In A Page
OB/GYN & Women's Health

Look for other books in this series!

In A Page Medicine

In A Page Pediatrics

In A Page Emergency Medicine

In A Page Surgery

In A Page Signs & Symptoms

In A Page Pediatric Signs & Symptoms

In A Page Neurology

In A Page
OB/GYN & Women's Health

Phyllis L. Carr, MD
Associate Dean of Students
Associate Professor of Medicine
Boston University School of Medicine
Boston, Massachusetts

Hope A. Ricciotti, MD
Assistant Professor, Obstetrics, Gynecology, and Reproductive Biology
OB/GYN Clerkship Director
Women's Health Education Theme Director
Harvard Medical School
Beth Israel Deaconess Medical Center
Boston, Massachusetts

Karen M. Freund, MD, MPH
Professor of Medicine
Boston University School of Medicine
Director, Center of Excellence in Women's Health
Boston University School of Medicine
Boston, Massachusetts

Scott Kahan, MD
Intern, Franklin Square Hospital
Baltimore, Maryland

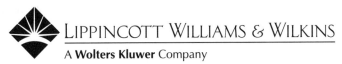

LIPPINCOTT WILLIAMS & WILKINS
A **Wolters Kluwer** Company
Philadelphia • Baltimore • New York • London
Buenos Aires • Hong Kong • Sydney • Tokyo

Printed in the United States of America

Library of Congress Cataloging-in-Publication Data

In a page OB/GYN & women's health / [edited by] Phyllis L. Carr ... [et al.].
    p. ; cm.
    Includes index.
    ISBN 1-4051-0380-9 (alk. paper)
        1. Obstetrics—Handbooks, manuals, etc.   2. Gynecology—Handbooks, manuals, etc.
        3. Women's health services—Handbooks, manuals, etc.
    I. Title: OB/GYN & women's health.   II. Carr, Phyllis L.

RG103.I5 2003
618—dc22

                                                                                2003045148

Acquisitions Editor: Donna Balado
Managing Editor: Kathleen Scogna
Marketing Manager: Emilie Linkins

The publishers have made every effort to trace the copyright holders for borrowed material. If they have inadvertently overlooked any, they will be pleased to make the necessary arrangements at the first opportunity.

To purchase additional copies of this book, call our customer service department at **(800) 638-3030** or fax orders to **(301) 223-2320**. International customers should call **(301) 223-2300**.

Visit Lippincott Williams & Wilkins on the Internet: http://www.LWW.com. Lippincott Williams & Wilkins customer service representatives are available from 8:30 am to 6:00 pm, EST.

06 07 08 09 10
2   3   4   5   6   7   8   9   10

Table of Contents

Table of Contents

Table of Contents

Table of Contents

Attributions

Alexandra Bageris
53. Upper Respiratory Tract Infections, 70. Deep Venous Thrombosis, 125. Heart Disease

Tracy A. Battaglia, MD, MPH
26. Breast Mass Evaluation

Marie Ellen Caggiano, MD
11. Contraception: Barrier Methods, 12. Contraception: Intrauterine Devices, 13. Contraception: Combination Hormonal Methods, 14. Contraception: Progestin-Only Methods, 27. Galactorrhea, 28. Vulvovaginitis, 30. Sexually Transmitted Diseases Overview, 31. Pelvic Inflammatory Disease, 32. Human Papilloma Virus, 33. Herpes Simplex Virus

Alison V. Cape, MD
46. Evaluation of an Abnormal Pap Smear, 47. Cervical Cancer, 85. Ectopic Pregnancy, 86. Hyperemesis Gravidarum, 87. Gestational Hypertenstion & Pre-eclampsia, 88. Cervical Incompetence

Andrea Charbonneau, MD, MSc
6. Adult Immunization, 7. Immunization During Pregnancy

Cynthia H. Chuang, MD
15. Emergency Contraception, 77. Domestic Violence

Donna Cohen, MD
56. Thyroid Disease, 57. Thyroid Disease in Pregnancy

Michele David, MD, MPH, MBA
64. Diabetes Mellitus, 66. Hypertension

Claudia De Young, MD, MSc
121. Osteoporosis

Elizabeth Dupuis, MD
124. Hormone Replacement Therapy

Matthew Freiberg, MD
60. Headache

Mary Gauthier-Delaplane, MD
17. Premenstrual Syndrome, 18. Abnormal Vaginal Bleeding, 19. Amenhorrea, 20. Dysmenorrhea & Pelvic Pain, 22. Polycystic Ovarian Syndrome, 23. Hisutism & Virilization, 24. Endometriosis & Adenomyosis, 37. Infertility, 38. Spontaneous & Recurrent Abortions, 39. Assisted Reproduction, 40. Abortion, 41. Sterilization (Male & Female)

Mary Beth Gordon, MD
79. Fetal Physiology, 91. Fetal Growth Restriction, 92. Macrosomia, 93. Oligohydramnios, 94. Polyhydramnios, 95. Hydrops Fetalis, 96. Intrauterine Fetal Demise, 97. Meconium Aspiration

Eric H. Green, MD, MSc
8. Breast Cancer Screening, 9. Cervical Cancer Screening

Melody Yen Hou, MD
82. Multiple Gestation, 89. Uterine Rupture, 90. Fetal Vessel Rupture, 103. Dystocia & the Augmentation of Labor, 108. Preterm Labor, 109. Preterm & Premature Rupture of Membranes, 110. Malpresentations

Attributions

Neda Laiteerapong
35. Toxic Shock Syndrome, 43. Breast Cancer, 52. Urinary Tract Infections

Janet F. McLaren, MD
25. Fibroids, 105. Episiotomy, 113. Normal Postpartum Care, 114. Postpartum Endometritis, 117. Mastitis

Omar Mulla-Ossman, MD
69. Epilespy, 126. Stroke

Daniel P. Newman, MD
54. Lower Respiratory Tract Infections, 55. Asthma, 58. Gallbladder Disease, 59. Irritable Bowel Syndrome, 72. Mitral Valve Prolapse

Mary Ellen Pavone, MD
29. Vulvar Disease, 61. Back Pain, 68. Obesity

Ngoc T. Phan
78. Maternal Physiology, 80. Prenatal Care, 81. Prenatal Diagnosis, 83. Bleeding in Early Pregnancy, 84. Bleeding in Late Pregnancy, 105. Episiotomy, 113. Normal Postpartum Care, 115. Postpartum Hemorrhage, 116. Post-Cesarean Wound Infection, 117. Mastitis

Amina Porter, BS
99. Initial Labor & Delivery Evaluation, 100. Fetal Heart Rate Monitoring, 101. Obstetrical Anesthesia, 102. Induction of Labor, 103. Dystocia & the Augmentation of Labor, 104. Vaginal & Operative Vaginal Delivery, 106. Cesarean Section Delivery, 107. Vaginal Birth After Cesarean Delivery, 111. Umbilical Cord Prolapse, 112. Shoulder Dystocia

Marion P. Russell, MD
1. Well Care of Female Adolescents, 2. Puberty, 3. Precocious Puberty, 4. Bulimia Nervosa, 5. Anorexia Nervosa, 62. Depression, 63. Anxiety Disorders, 118. Postpartum Depression

Michele Sinopoli, MD
10. Ovarian & Endometrial Cancer Screening, 34. Human Immunodeficiency Virus, 65. Diabetes in Pregnancy, 73. Tobacco Abuse, 74. Alcohol Abuse, 75. Substance Abuse, 76. Sexual Assault, 119. Well Care of Elderly Women, 120. Perimenopause

Tu-Mai Tran, MD
122. Urinary Incontinence, 123. Pelvic Prolapse

Christine M. Weeks, MD
42. Cancer in Pregnancy, 44. Solid Ovarian Tumors, 45. Epithilial Ovarian Carcinoma, 48. Uterine Cancer, 49. Vaginal Cancer, 51. Gestational Trophoblastic Neoplasia

Tiffany Jill Werbin, BSc, MA
36. Female Sexual Dysfunction

Jill Woods-Clay, MD
67. Chronic Hypertension in Pregnancy, 71. Thrombosis in Pregnancy

Abbreviations

5-FU	5-Fluorouracil		CPK	creatinine phosphate kinase
5HT	5-Hydroxytryptamine		CSE	combined spinal-epidural technique
β-hCG	beta subunit of human chorionic gonadotropin		CSF	cerebrospinal fluid
AC	abdominal circumference		CT	computerized tomography
ACA	anterior cerebral artery		CVA	costovertebral angle
ACE	angiotensin converting enzyme		CVS	chorionic villus sampling
ACOG	American College of Obstetricians and Gynecologists		D & C	dilation and curettage
			D & E	dilation and evacuation
ACTH	adrenal corticotrophic hormone		DCIS	ductal carcinoma in situ
ADH	antidiuretic hormone (vasopressin)		DES	diethylstilbestrol
AFI	amniotic fluid index		DEXA	dual-energy photon X-ray absorptiometry
AFP	alpha fetoprotein			
AGUS	atypical glandular cells of undetermined significance		DHEAS	dihydro-epiandrostene sulfate
			DIC	disseminated intravascular coagulation
AIDS	acquired immunodeficiency syndrome		dL	deciliter
			DM	diabetes mellitus
ALT	alanine aminotransferase		DNA	deoxyribonucleic acid
ANA	anti-nuclear antibody		DVT	deep venous thrombosis
ANC	absolute neutrophil count		DWI	diffusion weighted images
APA	anti-phospholipid (syndrome)		E. coli	Escherichia coli
APT	alum-precipitated toxoid		EBV	Epstein-Barr virus
AROM	artificial rupture of membranes		ECG	electrocardiogram
ASC-H	atypical squamous cells, cannot exclude HSIL		ECMO	extracorporeal membrane oxygenation
ASCUS	atypical squamous cells of undetermined significance		EDD	estimated date of delivery
			EE	ethinyl estradiol
AST	aspartate aminotransferase		EEG	electro-encephalogram
AutoPap	computer-assisted cytology interpretation system		EFW	estimated fetal weight
			EKG	electrocardiogram
BID	twice daily		ELISA	enzyme-linked immunosorbent assay
BMD	bone mineral density			
BMI	body mass index		EPDS	Edinburgh Postnatal Depression Scale
BP	blood pressure			
bpm	beats per minute		ERCP	endoscopic retrograde cholangiopancreatogram
BRCA1/2	breast cancer 1 and 2 genes			
BSO	bilateral salpingo-oophorectomy		ERT	estrogen replacement therapy
BUN	blood urea nitrogen		ESR	erythrocyte sedimentation rate
BV	bacterial vaginosis		FDA	Food and Drug Administration
CA-125	a tumor marker for ovarian cancer		FEV$_1$	forced expiratory volume in 1 second
Ca	cancer			
CAD	coronary artery disease		FHR	fetal heart rate
CAH	congenital adrenal hyperplasia		FSD	female sexual dysfunction
CBC	complete blood count		FSFI	female sexual function index
CDC	Centers for Disease Control		FSH	follicle-stimulating hormone
CHD	coronary heart disease		FVC	forced vital capacity
CHF	congestive heart failure		GABA	gamma-aminobutyric acid
CIN	cervical intra-epithelial neoplasia		GAD	generalized anxiety disorder
CMV	cytomegalovirus		GC	gonorrhea
CNS	central nervous system		GDM	gestational diabetes mellitus
COPD	chronic obstructive pulmonary disease		GI	gastrointestinal
			GIFT	gamete intrafallopian transfer
CPAP	continuous positive airway pressure		gm	gram
			GnRH	gonadotropin-releasing hormone

Abbreviations

GTN	gestational trophoblastic neoplasia	LSIL	low-grade squamous intra-epithelial lesion
GTT	glucose tolerance test	LV	left ventricle
GU	genitourinary	MAS	meconium aspiration syndrome
HAART	highly active antiretroviral therapy	MCA	middle cerebral artery
HbA$_{IC}$	glycosylated hemoglobin	MESA	microsurgical epididymal sperm aspiration
HBIG	hepatitis B immune globulin		
HC	head circumference	MI	myocardial infarction
hCG	human chorionic gonadotropin	mmHg	millimeters of mercury
HCT	hematocrit	MMI	methimazole
HDL	high-density lipoprotein	MMR	measles, mumps and rubella vaccine
HELLP	hemolysis, elevated liver functions, low platelets		
		MR	mitral regurgitation
HER-2neu	a receptor present in some breast cancers	MRA	magnetic resonance angiogram
		MRI	magnetic resonance imaging
HgbA$_{IC}$	glycosylated hemoglobin	MSAFP	maternal serum alpha fetoprotein
HGSIL	high-grade squamous intra-epitheilal lesion	MVP	mitral valve prolapse
		NEC	necrotizing enterocolitis
HIDA	hepatobiliary nuclear scan	NSAIDs	nonsteroidal anti-inflammatory drug(s)
HIV	human immunodeficiency virus		
HPF	high-power field	NTD	neural tube defect
HPV	human papilloma virus	OCD	obsessive-compulsive disorder
HR	heart rate	OCP	oral contraceptive pill
HRT	hormone replacement therapy	OPV	oral polio vaccine
HSIL	high-grade squamous intra-epithelial lesion	Pap	Papanicolaou smear
		PCOS	polycystic ovarian syndrome
HSV	herpes simplex virus	PCR	polymerase chain reaction
I:E ratio	inspiratory to expiratory ratio	PEG	percutaneous endoscopic gas-trostomy tube
IBS	irritable bowel syndrome		
ICSI	intracytoplasmic sperm injection	PF	peak flow
ICU	intensive care unit	PFTs	pulmonary function tests
IgG	immunoglobulins	PGD	pre-implantation genetic diagnosis
IM	intramuscular	PGE	prostaglandin
IPV	inactivated polio vaccine	PID	pelvic inflammatory disease
IVC	inferior vena cava	PMDD	premenstrual dysphoric disorder
IU	international units	PMNs	polymorphonuclear neutrophils
IUD	intrauterine device	PMS	premenstrual syndrome
IUFD	intrauterine fetal demise	PO	per os
IUGR	intrauterine growth restriction	POC	products of conception
IUI	intrauterine insemination	PPD	protein purified derivative
IV	intravenous	PRN	per nurse (or as needed)
IVF	in vitro fertilization	PROM	premature rupture of membranes
IVH	intraventricular hemorrhage	PTC	percutaneous transhepatic cholangiogram
LA	left atrium		
LDH	lactate dehydrogenase	PTL	preterm labor
LDL	low-density lipoprotein	PT/PTT	prothrombin time/partial thrombo-plastin time
LEEP	loop electrosurgical excision pro-cedure		
		PTSD	post-traumatic stress disorder
LFT	liver function test	PTU	propylthiouracil
LGA	large for gestational age	PVR	peripheral vascular resistance
LGSIL	low-grade squamous intra-epithelial lesion	QD	every day
		QID	four times daily
LGV	lymphogranuloma venereum	RBC	red blood cell
LH	luteinizing hormone	RDS	respiratory distress syndrome
LMP	last menstrual period	RNA	ribonucleic acid
LOC	loss of consciousness		

Abbreviations

ROM	rupture of membranes	TESA	testicular sperm extraction
RPR	rapid plasma reagin	TIA	transient ischemic attack
RSAB	recurrent spontaneous abortion	TID	three times daily
RSV	respiratory syncytial virus	TIG	tetanus immune globulin
RUQ	right upper quadrant	TMJ	temporomandibular joint
SAB	spontaneous abortion	TOA	tubo-ovarian abscess
SARS	sudden acute respiratory syndrome	TOL	trial of labor
SES	socioeconomic status	TRH	thyroid-releasing hormone
SGA	small for gestational age	TSH	thyroid-stimulating hormone
SHBG	steroidal hormone-binding globulin	TSS	toxic shock syndrome
SLE	systemic lupus erythematosis	TSST-1	toxic shock syndrome toxin–1
SSRI(s)	selective serotonin reuptake inhibitor(s)	TTE	transthoracic echocardiogram
		URI	upper respiratory infection
STD	sexually transmitted disease	U.S.	United States
T_3	thyroxine 3	UTI	urinary tract infection
T_4	thyroxine 4	VBAC	vaginal birth after cesarean
TAB	therapeutic abortion	VIN	vaginal intra-epithelial neoplasia
TAH	total abdominal hysterectomy	V/Q	ventilation-perfusion ratio
TBG	thyroid-binding globulin	VVC	vulvovaginal candidiasis
TCA(s)	tricyclic antidepressant(s)	VZIG	varicella zoster immune globulin
TCD	transcranial Doppler	WBC	white blood cell
Td	tetanus-diptheria	WHO	World Health Organization
TEE	transesophageal echocardiogram	XRT	radiation therapy
		ZIFT	zygote intrafallopian transfer

Contributors

Jesse D. Baer
Class of 2004
Drexel University College of Medicine
Philadelphia, Pennsylvania

Alexandra Bageris
Class of 2004
Boston University School of Medicine
Boston, Massachusetts

Tracy A. Battaglia, MD, MPH
Assistant Professor of Medicine
Boston University School of Medicine
Boston, Massachusetts

Marie Ellen Caggiano
Class of 2004
Boston University School of Medicine
Boston, Massachusetts

Alison V. Cape, MD
Intern, Obstetrics & Gynecology
Brigham and Women's Hospital
Massachusetts General Hospital
Boston, Massachusetts

Andrea Charbonneau, MD, MSc
Fellow, Section of General Internal Medicine
Boston Medical Center
Boston University School of Medicine
Boston, Massachusetts

Cynthia H. Chuang, MD
Fellow, Section of General Internal Medicine
Boston Medical Center
Boston University School of Medicine
Boston, Massachusetts

Donna Cohen, MD
Family Physician
Boston Medical Center
Boston, Massachusetts
Academic Fellow and Clinical Instructor
Department of Family Medicine
Boston University School of Medicine
Boston, Massachusetts

Michele David, MD, MPH, MBA
Co-Director, Haitian Health Institute at Boston Medical Center
Boston, Massachusetts
Assistant Professor of Medicine
Boston University School of Medicine
Boston, Massachusetts

Contributors

Claudia De Young, MD, MSc
Fellow, Section of General Internal Medicine
Boston Medical Center
Boston University School of Medicine
Boston, Massachusetts

Elizabeth Dupuis, MD
Assistant Professor of Medicine
Section of General Internal Medicine
Boston University School of Medicine
Boston Medical Center
Boston, Massachusetts
Chief, Women's Health Program
Quincy Medical Center
Quincy, Massachusetts

Matthew Freiberg, MD
Fellow, Section of General Internal Medicine
Boston Medical Center
Boston University School of Medicine
Boston, Massachusetts

Mary Gauthier-Delaplane, MD
Resident, General Surgery
Medical University of South Carolina
Charleston, South Carolina

Mary Beth Gordon, MD
Resident, Pediatrics
Children's Hospital
Boston, Massachusetts

Eric H. Green, MD, MSc
Fellow, Section of General Internal Medicine
Evans Department of Medicine
Boston Medical Center
Boston University School of Medicine
Boston, Massachusetts

Melody Yen Hou, MD
Resident, Obstetrics and Gynecology
University of California, Los Angeles Medical Center
Los Angeles, California

Neda Laiteerapong
Class of 2005
Boston University School of Medicine
Boston, Massachusetts

Janet F. McLaren, MD
Resident, Obstetrics & Gynecology
Brigham & Women's Hospital
Massachusetts General Hospital
Boston, Massachusetts

Contributors

Omar Mulla-Ossman, MD
Resident, Department of Neurology
Boston Medical Center
Boston, Massachusetts
Faculty Member
Boston University School of Medicine
Boston, Massachusetts

Daniel P. Newman, MD
Chief Resident, Internal Medicine
Boston Medical Center
Boston, Massachusetts
Clinical Instructor of Medicine
Boston University School of Medicine
Boston, Massachusetts

Alexis R. Palley
Class of 2003
Drexel University College of Medicine
Philadelphia, Pennsylvania

Mary Ellen Pavone, MD
PGY-1 Resident, OB/GYN
Johns Hopkins Hospital
Baltimore, Maryland

Ngoc T. Phan
Class of 2004
Harvard Medical School
Boston, Massachusetts

Amina Porter, BS
Class of 2004
Harvard Medical School
Boston, Massachusetts

Marion P. Russell, MD
Resident, Psychiatry
Harvard Longwood Program
Boston, Massachusetts

Michele Sinopoli, MD
Resident, Department of Obstetrics & Gynecology
University of Massachusetts Memorial Medical Center
Worcester, Massachusetts

Tu-Mai Tran, MD
Clinical Instructor of Family Medicine
Boston Medical Center
Boston, Massachusetts
Academic Fellow of Family Medicine
Boston University School of Medicine
Boston, Massachusetts

Contributors

Christine M. Weeks, MD
Resident, General Surgery
Brigham & Women's Hospital
Boston, Massachusetts

Tiffany Jill Werbin, BSc, MA
Class of 2004
Boston University School of Medicine
Boston, Massachusetts

Jill Woods-Clay, MD
Resident, Internal Medicine Department
Boston Medical Center
Boston, Massachusetts

Preface

In A Page OB/GYN & Women's Health is the fifth handbook of the *In A Page* series. The positive response to this series of books suggested the need for a more detailed text on obstetrics, gynecology, and women's health. This book continues the collaboration of healthcare providers at all levels—with authors ranging from advanced medical students to professors of medicine and obstetrics and gynecology.

Following the lead of the other books in the series, the popular one-page template to present a disease-per-page was used. This book also contains additional templates that allow reviews of screening, immunizations, contraception, and other preventive issues as well as labor and delivery topics. Due to the constraints of the size of the template and the need to keep each disease within a single page, the explanations and descriptions are succinct.

A special Attributions section has been added to the front matter of this book, to acknowledge the specific chapters written by each contributor. The number and title of each chapter they authored is listed in numerical order beneath the contributor's name.

Reviews from medical students and residents have been very positive. We anticipate that *In A Page OB/GYN & Women's Health* will be a valuable tool for looking up information quickly and concisely on rounds, as board review, and for independent study. We welcome any comments, questions, and suggestions. Please address correspondence to drkahan@yahoo.com.

Acknowledgments

We sincerely thank all contributors for their diligence on this project. Further, we must extend our deepest gratitude to the staff at Blackwell Publishing, especially Kate Heinle, Bev Copland, Deb Lally, and Laura DeYoung.

From Hope: My heartfelt thanks to the students at Harvard Medical School for their hard work on this manuscript, as well as their global commitment to education in women's health.

From Phyllis: I would like to thank Chris Blackburn for her assistance and patience in chapter preparation and the students of Boston University School of Medicine for their diligence, promptness, and enthusiasm for this book.

From Karen: I would like to thank the students, residents, and fellows of Boston University School of Medicine for their contributions and their dedication to addressing the healthcare needs of women.

From Scott: Thank you to Hope, Karen, Phyllis, and all contributors for your hard work on this project.

Adolescent Care

PHYLLIS L. CARR, MD
MARION P. RUSSELL, MD

Section 1

1. Well Care of Female Adolescents

- Most adolescent morbidity and mortality is attributable to preventable risk factors, making preventive services crucial to adolescent care
- The most prevalent causes of death are motor vehicle accidents, homicide, suicide, and unintentional injuries
- Factors that contribute to poor health include sedentary lifestyle, poor nutritional habits, smoking, substance abuse, reckless driving, unsafe sexual practices, and depression

Nutrition
- 30% of adolescent girls are overweight (BMI >25) and 15% are obese (BMI >30)
- Physical inactivity increases the risk of obesity, low self-esteem, depression, and substance abuse
- Poor nutrition also increases the risk of diabetes, hypertension, hypercholesterolemia, and coronary artery disease
- Obesity is preventable with proper nutritional counseling
- Adolescent girls are also at increased risk of eating disorders, including binge eating, bulimia, and anorexia
- Adequate calcium in adolescence is necessary to prevent osteoporosis in later years

Substance Use
- Adolescence is a time of experimentation with tobacco, alcohol, and illicit drugs
- Smoking is the most preventable risk factor for many causes of adult mortality
  –Peak age for initiating smoking is between 11 and 13; for initiating alcohol use is 12–15; and for marijuana use is about 14

Sexual Activity
- Adolescence is also a time of sexual exploration and identification
- Adolescent girls who drink or use drugs are more likely to have sexual intercourse and to do so without protection
- Half of 15–19 year old females have had sexual intercourse; only half of teen girls report using a condom
- About 20% of high school girls report physical or sexual abuse by a dating partner

Depression
- Adolescent girls are twice as likely as boys are to suffer from depression and are two to three times more likely to attempt suicide
- Adolescents who develop depression often have recurrences and a more severe course into adulthood
- Early detection and treatment are crucial to limit recurrences and morbidity

Evaluating the Adolescent
- The psychosocial history is the most important aspect of the interview
- Begin the interview with inquiries about innocuous topics, such as school, activities, and home life before moving on to more sensitive issues, such as depression, drugs, sexuality, and abuse
- Establish rules regarding confidentiality with the patient and family
- The adolescent should have the opportunity to meet with the provider separately from her parent or guardian
- The patient and parent or guardian should be made aware of circumstances in which confidentiality may be waived (e.g., if the patient is suicidal or is thought to be homicidal, or if the patient has experienced sexual or physical abuse, it must, by law, be reported; or if the patient has a life-threatening illness)
- The **HEADS** assessment is a structured screening tool for psychosocial issues
  –**H**ome - structure, stability, and safety of the home environment including family supports
  –**E**ducation - role of school in adolescent's life, including academic performance and attendance history
  –**A**ctivities, Affect, Ambition, Anger - hobbies, relationship with peers, physical activity, seat belt and bike helmet use, mood, thoughts about the future and important goals, risks of violence including homicidal ideation, access to firearms, history of physical abuse
  –**D**rugs - substance use or abuse by patient, family, or friends
  –**S**ex - sexual activity, sexual orientation, high-risk behaviors, history of sexual abuse or date rape

Examining the Adolescent
- The American Medical Association recommends an annual clinical visit throughout adolescence
- A comprehensive physical exam should be completed once during early adolescence (11–14 years), once during middle adolescence (15–17 years), and once in late adolescence (18–21 years)
  –This should include a blood pressure check, body mass index calculation, breast exam, height and weight measurements, and vital signs
  –If sexually active, patient should have annual pelvic exam with Pap smear and STD testing
  –Cholesterol screening should be done once during adolescence
  –Screening and guidance for issues identified in the **HEADS** assessment should also be provided

2. Puberty

Puberty is a transition period from childhood to adulthood that encompasses physical and emotional changes including further development of the genitals and secondary sex characteristics, ultimately leading to reproductive capability.
• The stages of puberty occur in a predictable sequence but the timing of and the initiation and velocity of change can vary widely among individuals
• In females, thelarche (breast buds) is usually the heralding sign of the onset of puberty followed by a height growth spurt, pubarche (appearance of pubic hair), and menarche (onset of menses)
• Puberty begins approximately 1 year earlier in females than males
• Thelarche occurs at an average age of 9 years with a normal range of 8–13 years
• The absence of secondary sex characteristics after age 13 merits investigation
• Asymmetry in breast development is not uncommon and should be observed until complete breast development has occurred around age 16–18 years
• The presence of hair in the axilla occurs at approximately age 12 and the onset of sebaceous secretion around age 13
• In general, peak height velocity immediately precedes onset of menarche, with an age range of 10–15 years and a mean age of 12 in girls
• Average age of menarche is 12.8 years; however, the normal age range is 10–16.5 years
• In general, menarche occurs 24 months after thelarche and relatively soon after peak height velocity
• Approximately 18 months is required between initial onset of menarche and regular ovulatory cycles

Developmental Stages
Tanner staging is used to stage the development of secondary sex characteristics
• Breast development
  –Stage 1: Preadolescent; elevation of papilla only
  –Stage 2: Breast bud; elevation of breast and papilla as small mound; enlargement of areolar diameter
  –Stage 3: Further enlargement and elevation of breasts and areola, with no separation of their contours
  –Stage 4: Projection of areola and papilla to form a secondary mound above the level of the breast
  –Stage 5: Mature stage; projection of papilla only due to recession of the areola to the general contour of the breast
• Pubic hair development
  –Stage 1: Preadolescent; vellus over pubes is not further developed than that over the abdominal wall (i.e., no pubic hair)
  –Stage 2: Sparse growth of long, slightly pigmented downy hair, straight or only slightly curled, appears along the labia
  –Stage 3: Considerably darker, coarser, and more curled; hair spreads sparsely over the junction of the pubes
  –Stage 4: Hair resembles adult in type, but the area covered by it is still considerably smaller than in the adult. There is no spread to the medial surface of the thighs
  –Stage 5: Adult in terms of quantity and type with distribution in horizontal pattern. Hair spreads to medial surface of thighs, but generally not up the linea alba (approximately 10% of women have public hair along the linea alba)

Psychosocial Issues to Address During Puberty and Adolescence
• Young adolescents are commonly preoccupied with physical changes because of rapid growth and development of secondary sex characteristics
• They may be concerned about deviation of growth from that of peers, especially excessively short or tall stature and delayed menses or breast development
• They are generally more comfortable with members of their own sex, and are developing curiosity about their sexuality
• They tend to be more attached to peers and shift their attention away from their family
• See **HEADS** assessment in *Well Care of Female Adolescents* entry

3. Precocious Puberty

Etiology/Pathophysiology

- Precocious puberty is defined as the appearance of physical and hormonal signs of pubertal development earlier than expected
  - Breast or pubic hair development before age 6 in black girls and age 7 in white girls
  - Menarche before age 10
  - Testicular enlargement >2.5 cm or pubic hair development before age 9 in boys
- Gonadotropin-dependent precocious puberty is defined by early maturation of the entire hypothalamic pituitary axis, accompanied by all of the physical and hormonal changes of puberty
  - More common in girls than boys
  - Usually idiopathic in girls (50–90%)
  - Often caused by CNS tumors in boys (50%)
- Gonadotropin-independent precocious puberty is very rare
  - May be seen with congenital adrenal hyperplasia; McCune-Albright syndrome; tumors of the adrenal glands, ovaries, or testes; and familial precocious puberty in boys

Differential Dx

- Premature thelarche (isolated appearance of breast development in girls <3 years of age)
- Premature pubarche (appearance of pubic hair without other signs of puberty in girls or boys younger than 7–8 years of age)

Presentation

- The earliest sign of puberty in girls is usually breast enlargement
- Enlargement of the clitoris
- Change in color of the vaginal mucosa from deep red to pale pink
- The earliest sign in boys is usually testicular enlargement; other signs include penile growth, reddening and thinning of the scrotum, and increased pubic hair

Diagnosis/Evaluation

- History and physical examination
- The diagnosis of gonadotropin-dependent precocious puberty is based on advanced bone age and pubertal hormonal levels
  - Elevated testosterone in boys
  - Elevated estradiol in girls
  - Random LH and FSH >5 IU/L is generally diagnostic for precocious puberty
  - Definitive diagnosis is confirmed by a brisk rise in LH (exceeding the rise in FSH) 20–40 minutes after infusion of GnRH
- Imaging studies may include radiographs of the hand and wrist to determine bone age
- MRI is often indicated in boys <9 years of age to evaluate for CNS pathology
- Pelvic ultrasound in girls will evaluate for ovarian tumors or cysts if gonadotropin-independent precocious puberty is suspected

Treatment

- Premature thelarche is benign and will resolve spontaneously
- Premature pubarche not caused by congenital adrenal hyperplasia is also benign and will resolve spontaneously
- Congenital adrenal hyperplasia is usually treated with oral contraceptive pills that contain low androgenic progesterone (e.g., levonorgestrel) or medroxyprogesterone with or without spironolactone to control hirsutism
- Gonadotropin-dependent precocious puberty is treated with injections of long-acting GnRH analogs (e.g., leuprolide acetate, nafarelin acetate)
- Follow up every 3–4 months to ensure the arrest of pubertal progression
- Monitor bone age yearly

Prognosis/Complications

- Normal adult height can be achieved in most cases if treatment is started before bone maturation becomes too advanced (generally before age 12 in girls and age 13 in boys)
- Significant improvement in adult height can be expected with treatment compared to predicted height at the start of therapy

4. Bulimia Nervosa

Etiology/Pathophysiology

- An eating disorder characterized by recurrent episodes of binge eating, lack of control over eating, purging behaviors, and persistent overconcern with body shape, weight, fasting, and/or excessive exercise
- Etiology is unknown; hypotheses include abnormal serotonergic functioning, abnormal satiety system functioning, and genetic predisposition
- 80% of bulimic patients are female; affects 1–4% of all females
- 15–20% of college-aged females engage in bulimic behaviors
- Onset peaks in late adolescence to early adulthood
- High rate of co-morbid disorders, including borderline personality disorder, depression, anxiety, and bipolar disorder
- Risk factors include a history of sexual abuse, personal or family history of substance abuse, and history of obesity, dieting, or depression

Differential Dx

- Major depressive disorder
- Anorexia nervosa
- Binge eating/purging
- Borderline personality disorder

Presentation

- Guilt about eating behaviors
- Abdominal pain and cramping
- Diarrhea secondary to laxative abuse
- Bloating
- Parotid gland enlargement
- Dental caries
- Calluses on knuckles
- Postural hypotension
- Muscle weakness and cramps secondary to hypokalemia

Diagnosis/Evaluation

- Recurrent binge eating followed by inappropriate compensatory behaviors to prevent weight gain, including self-induced vomiting, fasting, diuretic or laxative abuse, and excessive exercise
- Episodes occur at least 2 times per week for at least 3 months
- Feelings of loss of control accompany binges
- Undue emphasis on body shape and weight
- Purging type uses vomiting, laxatives, or diuretics
- Non-purging type uses exercise or fasting
- Patients are often normal weight or slightly overweight
- Obtain baseline vital statistics, including orthostatic blood pressures
- EKG may reveal signs of hypokalemia (e.g., U waves)
- Monitor regularly for electrolyte abnormalities (e.g., hypomagnesemia, hypocalcemia, hypophosphatemia) and to ascertain abstinence from purging

Treatment

- Medical stabilization, including correction of electrolyte disturbances and dehydration
- Monitor and stabilize electrolytes and magnesium as necessary
- Educate patients and family about complications such as dental caries, abdominal pain
- Nutritional rehabilitation (restore healthy eating habits)
- Cognitive behavioral therapy (individual, group, and family) and SSRIs (in weight-restored patients) have been shown to be effective

Prognosis/Complications

- 20% of affected patients continue to meet full diagnostic criteria 5–10 years after their initial presentation
- 50% of patients attain full recovery
- 30% relapse

5. Anorexia Nervosa

Etiology/Pathophysiology

- An eating disorder characterized by weight 15% below expected, amenorrhea, and either restriction of intake, bingeeating, or purging behavior
- The etiology of anorexia nervosa is unknown; hypotheses include genetic predispositions, psychodevelopmental difficulties, sociocultural influences, or neurochemical imbalances (e.g., serotonin)
- 95% of all anorexic patients are female; 1–3% of all females meet the diagnostic criteria for anorexia nervosa
- Onset peaks in late adolescence to early adulthood
- High rate of co-morbid disorders, including depression (present in 50–75% of cases), anxiety, and obsessive-compulsive disorder
- Risk factors include a family history of disordered eating or mental illness, early puberty, weight dissatisfaction, a drive for perfection, dieting, and low self-esteem
- The athletic triad commonly afflicts female athletes and consists of disordered eating, amenorrhea, and osteoporosis (and often excessive exercise), but does not meet the full criteria for anorexia nervosa

Differential Dx

- Major depressive disorder
- Thyroid disease
- Inflammatory bowel disease
- Malabsorption syndromes
- Bulimia nervosa
- Body dysmorphic disorder

Presentation

- Weight loss
- Fatigue
- Amenorrhea
- Abdominal pain
- Intolerance to cold
- Hair loss
- Fainting spells
- Lanugo (fine hair on face/body)
- Bone pain secondary to stress fractures
- Hypothermia

Diagnosis/Evaluation

- Defined weight loss or failure to gain weight during growth, leading to body weight <85% of expected
- Excessive fear of gaining weight or being obese
- Distorted body image
- Interruption of menses for at least 3 consecutive months
- Restricting type: Limits calorie intake
- Purging type: Self-induced vomiting, laxative abuse, diuretic use
- Obtain baseline vital statistics, including orthostatic blood pressures
- EKG may reveal changes consistent with hypokalemia (e.g., U waves), bradycardia, and prolonged QT interval with risk of sudden death
- Electrolyte monitoring (potassium, magnesium, phosphorus) is necessary to evaluate for hypokalemia, metabolic alkalosis, hypophosphatemia, hypocalcemia, and hypomagnesemia
- Bone density testing to detect osteopenia/osteoporosis

Treatment

- Hospitalization is indicated if weight is <70–75% of ideal body weight, if the patient has persistent suicidality, or with failure of outpatient treatment
- Weight restoration via a structured eating program
- Individual, group, or family therapy
- SSRIs have been shown to be effective (in weight-restored patients)
- Prevention and treatment of osteoporosis

Prognosis/Complications

- >10% mortality
- 30–50% fully recover
- 80% partly recover
- Nearly 50% of patients develop concurrent bulimic symptoms

Gynecologic & Preventive Care

Section 2

MARIE ELLEN CAGGIANO
PHYLLIS L. CARR, MD
ANDREA CHARBONNEAU, MD, MSc
CYNTHIA H. CHUANG, MD
KAREN M. FREUND, MD, MPH
ERIC H. GREEN, MD, MSc
MICHELE SINOPOLI, MD

6. Adult Immunization

Indications

- Influenza: Administered yearly (autumn); recommended for those >50, healthcare workers, nursing home residents, high-risk persons' housemates
- Pneumococcus: One dose for immunocompetent persons >65; revaccination after age 65 for those with cardiac, pulmonary, or liver disease; diabetes; CSF leak; immunocompromise (including those with splenic dysfunction); and long-term care residents
- Tetanus-diphtheria (Td): Toxoid, recommended every 10 years universally
- Hepatitis B: Three-dose vaccine recommended for adults at risk of exposure (e.g., intravenous drug use, healthcare workers, multiple sexual partners, travelers, immunocompromised, dialysis patients)
- Hepatitis A: Two-dose vaccine recommended for those at exposure risk (e.g., travelers, daycare workers, chronic liver disease, food handlers)
- Measles-mumps-rubella (MMR): Two-dose vaccine for those susceptible to exposure (e.g., fertile women, college students, healthcare workers, international travelers); one-dose vaccine for other adults born after 1957
- Varicella: Two-dose vaccine for those susceptible and without documented immunity (e.g., healthcare workers, fertile women, travelers, teachers, military, correctional facilities)

Epidemiology

- About 45% of the population >65 years and 12% of those susceptible between ages 18–49 are immunized against pneumococcus
- About 64% of those >65 and 20% of those susceptible between ages 18–49 are immunized against influenza
- There is waning immunity to diphtheria and tetanus among adults (47% immune)

Side Effects

- Safety: True contraindications are rare; may include severe hypersensitivity reactions (anaphylaxis, neurologic sequelae)
- Local tenderness at administration site, low-grade temperature, and malaise can occur with all vaccines
- Rare association of Guillain-Barré syndrome with influenza vaccine
- Those with history of anaphylaxis to eggs or neomycin should avoid MMR
- Oral polio vaccine (OPV), a live vaccine, has been associated with paralytic disease; it has been discontinued in the U.S., except in children traveling to endemic areas within 4 weeks

Alternative Treatments

- Influenza: Amantadine 200 mg QD until 24–48 hours after symptom resolution
- Pneumococcus: Antimicrobial treatment for pneumonia for 14 days (e.g., fluoroquinolone, cephalosporin)
- Td: Post-exposure to tetanus—clean wounds, administer Td and TIG (tetanus immune globulin); post-exposure to diphtheria—antitoxin, 14-day course of penicillin
- Hepatitis B: HBIG and vaccine series following exposure; 1-year course of lamivudine or 6–24 months of interferon-α for disease
- Hepatitis A: Hepatitis A gamma globulin for one dose (protective if within 2 weeks of exposure)
- MMR: Measles post-exposure—immunoglobulin followed 6 months later by MMR vaccine (protective if within 6 days of exposure)
- Varicella: Post-exposure, consider vaccine; post-exposure for pregnant or immunocompromised, use VZIG; acyclovir, famciclovir, or valacyclovir may be used for severe cases

Efficacy

- Less immunogenicity of varicella vaccine among adults; about 27% report mild breakthrough cases (far lower among children)
- There is waning immunity 5 years after pneumococcal vaccination, but the role of re-administration in the general population unclear (efficacy estimated at 70% in elderly)
- Efficacy of influenza vaccine among elderly is estimated at 35–65%
- Efficacy of hepatitis A and B vaccines is estimated at >95% if the full course is administered; long-term seroprotection is still unknown
- Population-based studies consider cost effectiveness of vaccine administration as well as vaccine efficacy (measured by comparing number of disease cases among vaccinated compared with unvaccinated persons)

Complications

- Avoid administration of MMR and varicella for at least 5 months after administration of immune globulin (reduced vaccine efficacy in presence of passive antibodies); if MMR or varicella is given first, hold immune globulin administration for 2 weeks
- Pneumococcus is the leading cause of vaccine-preventable death in the U.S.
- For more information, contact the CDC immunization hotline at 800-232-2522 or www.cdc.gov

7. Immunization During Pregnancy

Indications

- Pneumococcus: Should be given in the second or third trimesters to women at high risk for pneumococcal infection (cardiac, pulmonary, or liver disease; immunocompromise; diabetes)
- Hepatitis B: Should be administered to gravidas completing an immunization series begun prior to conception and to non-immune women at exposure risk
- Hepatitis A: Little information on use in pregnancy, but as with other inactivated vaccines, the risk is presumed to be low
- Tetanus-diphtheria (Td): Should be administered to pregnant women who have not completed the 3-dose primary immunization or 10-year booster
- Influenza: Should be administered from Oct. to mid-Nov. for gravid women with chronic medical conditions, regardless of pregnancy stage; all others should be immunized during the second or third trimester
- MMR: Contraindicated in pregnancy because of theoretical risk of congenital rubella syndrome, although there has never been a reported case from inadvertent vaccination in pregnancy
- Varicella: Contraindicated in pregnancy because of theoretical risk of fetal varicella infection, although there has never been a reported case

Epidemiology

- Preconception planning and vaccination prior to pregnancy
- Routine immunization during pregnancy should be delayed until the second or third trimester because of teratogenicity concerns

Side Effects

- Although non-live vaccines can be administered safely to non-immune women during pregnancy, the ideal time to immunize is prior to conception
- Live vaccines are contraindicated in pregnancy unless imminent danger of exposure (e.g., yellow fever); pregnancy should be avoided for 28 days following the administration of live vaccines (varicella, MMR)
- Inadvertent vaccination with varicella or MMR is *not* an indication for abortion

Alternative Treatments

- See also *Adult Immunization* entry; drug-specific pregnancy safety classification is reviewed there
- Amantadine (influenza) is a pregnancy class C drug (may have teratogenic effects, no controlled studies in humans)
- Fluoroquinolones are pregnancy class C drugs
- Cephalosporins are pregnancy class B drugs (no teratogenic effects noted in controlled human studies)
- Immunoglobulins are pregnancy class C drugs
- Lamivudine (hepatitis B) is a pregnancy class C drug
- Acyclovir (varicella) and all of the antiviral DNA polymerase inhibitors are pregnancy class B drugs

Efficacy

- Refer to *Adult Immunization* entry
- Pregnancy does not alter the efficacy of any vaccine

Complications

- Poliomyelitis: Oral polio vaccine (OPV), a live vaccine, has been associated with paralytic disease; it has been discontinued in the U.S., except in children traveling to endemic areas within 4 weeks; traveling gravidas should receive a booster with inactivated polio vaccine (IPV) if immunized in the past, and a primary IPV schedule if nonimmunized (see CDC link below)
- For more information, refer to the CDC immunization hotline 800-232-2522 or www.cdc.gov/nip/

8. Breast Cancer Screening

Indications

- Mammography every 1–2 years beginning at age 40 is recommended by almost all North American public health groups
- In patients with a first-degree relative (mother or sister) with breast cancer, begin mammography 5 years before the age of disease in the youngest affected family member
- There is some controversy regarding mammography in women 40–49 years of age due to fewer women studied in the randomized controlled trials and borderline significance in the apparent benefit
- There is also controversy regarding mammography in women older than 70 years, as this group was not included in the trials
- Mammography is generally continued until co-morbid illness nullifies any benefit from continued screening
- Although breast cancer is more common in older women, younger women have the most years to gain from early detection

Epidemiology

- Previous history of breast cancer
- History of radiation therapy to the chest
- Older age: Proven mortality benefit from randomized control trials for age >50
- Unlikely to have a beneficial effect on mortality in women with an estimated life expectancy ≤10 years
- Mammography works best in postmenopausal women without HRT

Side Effects

- Pain from compression of the breast during mammography
- Anxiety, pain, morbidity, and rare mortality from the evaluation of false positives

Alternative Treatments

- No screening: Some have argued that breast cancer screening is not proven to be effective, primarily due to the poor quality of early trials and the lack of evidence that breast cancer screening of any type reduces all cause mortality
- Clinician breast exam: Often recommended to be used in conjunction with mammography but are not considered to be sufficient for screening without concurrent mammography
- Self breast exam: Self breast exams lead to more discovered masses but have not been proven to reduce mortality from breast cancer; thus, they are not considered to be sufficient for breast cancer screening
- New radiographic screening techniques (e.g., MRI) are under development
- Genetic testing for BRCA1 and 2 genes should be considered in patients with a strong family history of breast and/or ovarian cancer

Efficacy

- Sensitivity is 71–98%
- Sensitivity is highest in older women
- Mammography will miss 1 in 4 breast cancers in women aged <50
- Specificity is 94–97%
- At least 80% of positive mammograms will be false positives (no cancer will be found)
- Meta-analysis of randomized, controlled trials suggests a statistically significant 15–30% reduction in breast cancer mortality over 14 years with mammography; this trend is true in younger and older women

Complications

- Treatment of DCIS lumpectomy/XRT or mastectomy despite its uncertain prognosis
- Rarely, induction of breast cancer may occur secondary to screening (<8 deaths/1,000,000 person-years of annual screening)

9. Cervical Cancer Screening

Indications

- Most groups recommend an annual Pap smear for all women after becoming sexually active or at age 18
- Most groups recommend that low-risk women (those with three consecutive normal Pap smears and no history of abnormal pap smears) can have Pap smears every 2–3 years
- Pap smears should be discontinued in women who have had a total abdominal hysterectomy for benign conditions
- Some groups recommend that Pap smears can be discontinued at age 65–70 in low-risk women who have had multiple recent normal Pap smears, others recommend continued lifetime screening every 2–3 years
- Vaccination against HPV has been shown effective against persistent infection and cytologic abnormalities for the most common (HPV type 16); vaccination will likely change protocols on screening in the future

Epidemiology

- HPV infection thought to be causative agent
- Additional risk factors
  - HIV infection or other immunosuppression
  - Early first intercourse
  - Multiple lifetime sexual partners
  - History of STDs
  - Radiation exposure
  - Smoking
  - Low SES
  - "High-risk" sexual partner
- Peak age CIN: late 20s
- Peak age Ca in situ: 35
- Peak age cancer: 55–60

Side Effects

- Discomfort associated with speculum examination in order to obtain the test
- Discomfort may be significant with
  - Vaginismus
  - Mucosal atrophy
  - Intact hymenal ring
  - History of sexual trauma/abuse
- Minimal vaginal bleeding with normal cervix

Alternative Treatments

- AutoPap: Computer-assisted interpretation of standard Pap smears (compared to manual inspection) used for 2nd reads
- Liquid-based Pap: The sample is collected in standard fashion, but placed in liquid preservative; the laboratory prepares the slide and is able to separate cervical cells from other cells, resulting in improved adequacy to the smear; liquid can be later used for HPV DNA testing
- Visual inspection of the cervix: Effective as an adjunct to Pap smear but not generally considered sufficient for screening
- Cervicoscopy: Inspection of the cervix after acetic-acid wash may be used in areas where Paps are not available (usually 3rd world countries); combining with photography (cervicography) and magnification (speculoscopy) may have higher sensitivity and specificity but are still under development
- HPV testing: Since most HPV infections are transient, screening for HPV is not an effective tool; HPV screening is useful in triage of ASCUS (see *Evaluation of an Abnormal Pap Smear* entry)

Efficacy

- Considered the most successful cancer detection and prevention strategy ever developed
- Observational studies have shown a marked decrease in the incidence of invasive cervical cancer with its use
- Although sensitivity of a single test is low (60–80% for high-grade lesions), the combination of repeat screening and the long time period of progression from CIN to invasive cancer makes the test very effective
- Specificity is >90% for high-grade lesions
- In women with a history of normal Pap smears, on a single screen <10 cases of high-grade abnormalities (HGSIL or cancer) will be found for every 10,000 women screened
- In this group, only 1 of every 34 women with HSIL on Pap will actually have HSIL or cancer on further evaluation

Complications

- Further necessary testing and biopsies for false positive results
- Psychological distress and possible unnecessary treatment for women with low-grade abnormalities (which may regress spontaneously)

10. Ovarian & Endometrial Cancer Screening

Indications

- Currently, ovarian and endometrial cancer screening is not recommended for average risk women
- Factors that modify the risk of ovarian cancer
  - Nulliparity, first birth after age 35, and infertility may increase the risk of ovarian cancer
  - Pregnancy *reduces* the risk of ovarian cancer by 25–50%
  - Oral contraceptive pills *reduce* the risk of ovarian cancer by 35%
- Most endometrial cancers are due to excess unopposed estrogen
  - Tamoxifen (a partial agonist), estrogen replacement therapy, obesity, anovulation, and estrogen secreting tumors are sources
  - 1 in 1000 risk of endometrial cancer for postmenopausal women not on ERT; becomes 1 in 100 for those on unopposed postmenopausal estrogens
  - A woman with postmenopausal bleeding is at increased risk for endometrial cancer
- Familial syndromes that increase the risk of both ovarian and endometrial cancers
  - Breast-ovarian cancer syndrome (BRCA1 or BRCA2 gene mutation)
  - Lynch II syndrome (colon, breast, endometrium, and ovarian cancer)

Epidemiology

- Ovarian cancer
  - Leading cause of death from a gynecologic malignancy in U.S.
  - 1.4% lifetime incidence
  - 90% survival for stage I disease; 20% survival for clinically advanced disease
- Endometrial cancer
  - Most common gynecologic malignancy in U.S.
  - 95% survival for stage I disease; 26% for stages III/IV

Side Effects

- Physical discomfort from bimanual exam and ultrasound
- Cramping and pain from endometrial biopsy
- Anxiety due to exam and waiting for results

Alternative Treatments

- Other than yearly bimanual pelvic exam and Pap smear, screening is not currently recommended for ovarian and endometrial cancer in the average woman
- Ovarian cancer
  - Screen for tumor marker CA-125, which is associated with ovarian cancer, can be done for high-risk patients
  - Pelvic ultrasound to detect ovarian masses can be done for patients at high risk of ovarian cancer
- Endometrial cancer
  - Transvaginal ultrasound demonstrating an endometrial thickness ≤5 mm in a postmenopausal woman is a strong negative predictor for cancer
  - Endometrial biopsy for peri- and postmenopausal bleeding or AGUS on Pap smear
- Pap smear
  - High-risk syndromes
  - Any endometrial or glandular cell on Pap smear in post-menopausal women

Efficacy

- Pelvic exams and Pap smears are neither sensitive nor specific for endometrial or ovarian cancer
- Serum CA-125 levels are elevated in over 80% of women with ovarian cancer
  - 50% sensitivity for stage I disease; 90% sensitivity for stage II disease
  - 99% specificity (also elevated in endometrial, breast, and lung cancers; endometriosis; benign ovarian cysts; and normally elevated in 1% of healthy women)
- Pelvic ultrasound
  - 85% sensitivity for detecting ovarian cancer
  - 94% specificity for detecting ovarian cancer
- Endometrial biopsy
  - 88–97% sensitivity for detecting cancer in patients with postmenopausal bleeding
  - Detects only 1.7 endometrial carcinomas per 1000 person-years in asymptomatic postmenopausal women

Complications

- The incidence and prevalence of ovarian cancer are low, making a false positive screening test more likely
- Prophylactic salpingo-oophorectomy for those with BRCA mutations
  - Mechanism of benefit through estrogen and progesterone deficiency
- Risk of surgical complications
- Psychological morbidity
- Possible infection from endometrial biopsy

11. Contraception: Barrier Methods

Indications

- Any sexually active person at risk for STDs should use condoms (latex and polyurethane are protective against viral transmission; condoms made from animal membranes are not)
- Persons with a history of transmissible diseases (herpes, HPV, hepatitis B/C, HIV) should use condoms to prevent infection of their partners
- Adolescents are at higher risk for STD infection and unwanted pregnancy and should be advised to use condoms in addition to another method
- Barrier methods are useful in women who do not want or cannot take hormones
- Women who are willing and able to insert the device prior to intercourse may use cervical caps and diaphragms; the initial fitting must be done by a clinician; these do not protect against STDs
- Spermicides are available as creams, foams, sponges, suppositories, and jellies; they may be used alone, but are more effective when added to another barrier method
    - Spermicides may decrease transmission of certain STDs but do not prevent the transmission of HIV

Epidemiology

- Effective barriers include condoms (male and female), vaginal diaphragm, and cervical cap
- Addition of spermicide to above methods increases efficacy
- Condoms are the only available method to prevent transmission of STDs, and all persons at risk should be advised to use condoms in addition to other methods

Side Effects

- Some people complain of decreased sexual pleasure when using condoms
- Recurrent UTIs may occur with use of cervical cap or diaphragm, and less frequently with the female condom
- Spermicides may cause irritation and/or hypersensitivity in either partner

Alternative Treatments

- Hormonal methods
- IUD
- Natural methods (high failure rate)
- Tubal ligation/vasectomy (if permanent contraception is desired)

Efficacy

- 1-year failure rates with male condoms are 2% with perfect use and 15% with typical use; rates for female condoms are 5% and 20%, respectively
    - Condoms should be promptly removed and discarded after ejaculation has occurred; they may not be reused
    - Only water-based lubricants should be used with condoms, as petroleum or oil-based formulas can cause tears
- Cervical caps are more effective in nulliparous women (16% 1-year failure rate vs 32% in multiparous women)
- Diaphragms are slightly more effective, regardless of parity
    - 6% 1-year failure rate with perfect use
    - 16% 1-year failure rate with typical use
- Spermicide must be used with caps and diaphragms
    - Spermicide alone has a failure rate of 30%

Complications

- Condoms made from latex may cause allergic reactions (2–3% of the population is latex-sensitive); cervical caps are also made from latex
- If condom breaks or slips, emergency contraception should be offered; some clinicians provide patients with an emergency contraceptive prescription to keep on hand
- Toxic shock syndrome may be associated with cervical caps and diaphragms if left in the vagina for prolonged periods of time (rare)
- Improperly fitted caps and diaphragms can cause trauma to the cervix and vagina
- Men and women may develop allergies to spermicides

12. Contraception: Intrauterine Devices

Indications

- An IUD is inserted into the endometrial cavity to prevent pregnancy
- For women under the following circumstances
  - Desire long-term reversible contraception
  - At low risk for STDs (mutually monogamous relationship)
  - With no history of pelvic inflammatory disease
  - With medical contraindications to or side effects with estrogen use
- Levonorgestral-containing IUDs are used for the treatment of menorrhagia/dysmenorrhea and to protect against endometrial carcinoma in women taking hormone replacement who cannot tolerate oral progestins
- Contraindications
  - Pregnancy
  - Undiagnosed abnormal uterine bleeding
  - Untreated lower genital tract infections
  - Malignancies of the genital tract
  - Multiple sexual partners (IUDs do not protect against STDs)
  - Immunocompromise
  - For Copper T: Wilson's disease or copper allergy
  - Acute PID or endometritis

Epidemiology

- Intrauterine devices are the most commonly used method of contraception worldwide; however, in the U.S. <1% of women choose an IUD
- Two IUDs are currently available in the U.S.: Paraguard Copper T and Mirena, which releases levonorgestrel
- IUDs must be inserted and removed by a clinician
- Cost $300–400

Side Effects

- Copper T:
  - Menorrhagia (monthly bleeding increased by 35%)
  - Dysmenorrhea
  - Discomfort at insertion
  - Vaginitis
- Mirena:
  - Amenorrhea (20% by 1 year, 60% by 5 years)
  - Spotting and irregular bleeding
  - Headaches
  - Acne
  - Breast tenderness
  - Discomfort at insertion
  - Vaginitis

Alternative Treatments

- Hormonal methods
- Barrier methods
- Natural methods (high failure rate)
- Tubal ligation/vasectomy (if permanent contraception is desired)
- IUD insertion post-coitally as emergency contraception

Efficacy

- Copper T lasts for 10 years
  - Mechanism of action is two-fold: Copper is spermicidal, and a sterile inflammatory response is triggered in the endometrium
  - <1% 1-year failure rate
  - 2–3% cumulative 10-year failure rate
- Mirena lasts for 5 years
  - Sperm motility is impaired by changes in cervical mucus and uterotubal fluid; the endometrium is unfavorable to implantation
  - Some women may become anovulatory (5–15%)
  - 0.1% 1-year failure rate
  - 0.7% cumulative 5-year failure rate

Complications

- Uterine perforation (1/1000), surgically remove IUD (usually via laparoscopy)
  - Occurs at insertion
  - Pain, vaginal bleeding, rapid pulse
  - Remove IUD; use other contraception
- Pelvic inflammatory disease (1/1000)
  - Occurs around time of insertion
  - Risk higher with untreated lower genital tract infections
  - Antibiotics; remove IUD if no response
- Missing strings
  - Locate with ultrasound or X-ray
- Expulsion (occurs first month after insertion)
  - Rule out pregnancy
  - Replace (if desired)
- Pregnancy: Confirm intrauterine pregnancy; remove IUD (higher risk of miscarriage)

13. Contraception: Combination Hormonal Methods

Indications

- Healthy, reproductive-aged women who desire contraception
- For treatment of common gynecologic problems including endometriosis, dysmenorrhea, PCOS, functional ovarian cysts, and iron deficiency anemia
- Teenagers may be good candidates; however, it is important to counsel them to continue using condoms for protection against STDs (combination hormonal contraceptives do not protect against STDs)
- Health benefits include
  - Regulation of menses with decreased bleeding
  - Decreased dysmenorrhea and physical symptoms of PMS
  - Decreased risk of epithelial ovarian cancer
  - Decreased risk of endometrial cancer
  - Decreased risk of benign breast disease
  - Reduced rates of PID and ectopic pregnancy
  - Protects against loss of bone density
- Contraindications include a history of thromboembolic disease or estrogen-dependent cancer, smoking, uncontrolled hypertension, hepatic adenoma, significant hepatic dysfunction, and undiagnosed vaginal bleeding

Epidemiology

- Hormones (estrogen and progestin) suppress ovulation, thicken cervical mucus, and atrophy the endometrial lining
- Most combinations use ethinyl estradiol (EE) as the estrogen
- Currently available combinations use "low-dose" formulas (20–35 μg EE)
- Delivery route may be via pill, transdermal patch, vaginal ring, or injectable depot (Lunelle)

Side Effects

- Spotting, especially first few cycles
- Headache, migraines may worsen
- Nausea (rarely vomiting), especially first few cycles
- Bloating and weight gain (not a substantial difference than in non-users)
- Hepatic adenoma (increased in combos using ≥50 μg of estrogen)
- Elevation of blood pressure (1% will develop significant hypertension which is reversible if hormones are discontinued)
- Amenorrhea may occur with "continuous use"; however, this may be useful in women with heavy and/or painful menses

Alternative Treatments

- Progestin-only hormonal
- Intrauterine device
- Barrier methods
- Natural methods (high failure rate)
- Tubal ligation/vasectomy (if permanent contraception is desired)

Efficacy

- 1-year failure rates for oral formulations
  - Perfect use: 0.3%
  - Typical use: 4–6%
  - Key to success is that the patient must be able to take a pill every day
- 1-year failure rates for transdermal patch
  - Perfect use: 0.3–0.6%
  - Studies have shown better compliance vs pills
  - May be less effective in obese women
- 1-year failure rates for monthly injectables: 0.05–3%
- Vaginal ring: Failure rate of 0.65% per 100 woman-years (all occur within first year)
- Certain medications (e.g., antibiotics, anticonvulsants) may reduce efficacy of hormonal methods; women should be counseled to use a backup method while taking these medications (these are theoretical risks; however, there are no actual data)

Complications

- Venous thromboembolism
  - 10–30/100,000 vs 4–8/100,000 in non-users
  - Risk is lower than in pregnancy
  - Risk further increased in factor V Leiden and protein S or C abnormalities (prior screening is not indicated before OCP use)
- MI and stroke
  - Women at risk are smokers over 35
  - All users should be counseled to stop smoking and control modifiable risk factors for cardiovascular disease
- Breast cancer
  - Current research does NOT show that combination oral contraceptives increase the risk of breast cancer, but there is controversy if a first-degree relative has breast cancer or if BRCA1 or 2 positive

14. Contraception: Progestin-Only Methods

Indications

- Progestin implants thicken cervical mucus and have variable effects on ovulation
- Health benefits of progestin-only methods are similar to the combination hormonal methods, with the exception of protection against bone loss
- Indicated for women with a history of thromboembolism or risk factors for cardiovascular disease (i.e., those who cannot take estrogen)
- Indicated in women who desire a rapidly reversible method of contraception
- Progestins are useful in lactating women, as they have no effect on quantity of milk or infant weight gain
- Candidates for progestins must be reliable pill-takers, as pills must be taken at the same time every day; a delay of more than 3 hours is equivalent to a missed pill, as the effect on cervical mucus lasts only 27 hours
- Depo-Provera is indicated in women who desire intermediate to long-term contraception (return to baseline fertility averages 10 months)
  - Depo-Provera is a useful method in adolescents, and its introduction in the U.S. has been credited with a reduction in the teen pregnancy rate
- None of the progestin-only methods protect against STDs

Epidemiology

- Progestin pills (mini-pills) contain only a progestin and are taken daily with no hormone-free intervals
- Depo-Provera injections are administered every 3 months
- Progestin-containing implants (such as Norplant) are placed in the subcutaneous tissue and offer contraception for 3–5 years; however, they are currently not available in the U.S.

Side Effects

- Progestins are associated with a high degree of irregular bleeding; amenorrhea in 10% of patients
- Depo-Provera injections are associated with irregular bleeding, especially during the first few months
  - 50% have amenorrhea by 1-year, 80% by 5 years
  - Also associated with hot flashes, decreased libido, vaginal dryness, hair loss, mood swings, headaches, and acne
  - Progressive weight gain with an average of 5.4 lbs in the first year and 16 lbs by 5 years
- Side effects associated with implants are similar to those of Depo-Provera; however, there may be less weight gain

Alternative Treatments

- Combination hormonal (if estrogen not contraindicated)
- Barrier methods
- IUD
- Natural methods (high failure rate)
- Tubal ligation/vasectomy (for permanent contraception)

Efficacy

- Progestin-only pills
  - Thickened cervical mucus prevents sperm from passing into the uterus; 50% women remain ovulatory
  - 0.3% 1-year failure rate with perfect use
  - 8% 1-year failure rate with typical use
- Depo-Provera injections
  - Suppresses ovulation, thickens cervical mucus, thins endometrium
  - 0.3% 1-year failure rate if injections are taken on time
  - Half of users will discontinue within first year because of side effects

Complications

- The most common complication is pregnancy (due to noncompliance with pill regimen)
- Depo-Provera injections
  - Severe allergic reactions may rarely occur after injection
  - Increased risk for diabetes in breast-feeding women who had gestational diabetes

15. Emergency Contraception

Indications

- Reduces risk of pregnancy when initiated within 72 hours after unprotected intercourse
- If last menstrual period is >4 weeks ago or there have been other episodes of unprotected intercourse since the last menstrual period, then pregnancy testing may be indicated before initiating emergency contraception
- May be prescribed during routine health maintenance visits for the patient to have on hand in advance of need
- If the patient has known contraindication to estrogen (e.g., estrogen hypersensitivity, hypertension, breast cancer, history of thromboembolic disease), a progestin-only method is recommended
- Mechanism of action: Prevents pregnancy most likely by interfering with ovulation—NOT an abortifacient
- The first dose is taken within 72 hours of unprotected intercourse; the second dose is taken 12 hours later; current FDA approved regimens for emergency contraceptive pills contain levonorgestrel 0.75 mg per dose (progestin-only method) or ethinyl estradiol 100 μg and levonorgestrel 0.50 mg per dose (combined estrogen-progestin method)

Epidemiology

- Consider emergency contraception for all women of reproductive age for any of the following situations
  - Failure to use contraceptive method
  - Backup to barrier contraception
  - Known contraceptive failure (e.g., condom breakage, incorrect pill use)
  - Rape/sexual assault

Side Effects

- Nausea/vomiting: 16%/6% with progestin-only method and 42%/23% with combined estrogen-progestin method (taking oral meclizine prior to first dose significantly reduces nausea and vomiting with combined method)
- Altered next menses: May be earlier or later than expected, but should perform pregnancy testing if no menses within 1 week of expected time
- Abdominal cramping
- Breast tenderness
- Irregular vaginal spotting or bleeding
- Dizziness, fatigue, headache
- Side effects may last for a few days, but generally resolve within 24 hours

Alternative Treatments

- Emergency IUD insertion within 7 days of unprotected intercourse (failure rate <0.1%)
- "Wait and see"—if no menses when expected, perform pregnancy testing

Efficacy

- 85% risk reduction of pregnancy with progestin-only methods
- 74% risk reduction of pregnancy with combined estrogen-progestin methods

Complications

- No reported adverse events when inadvertently given to a woman who is already pregnant
- No increase in risk of teratogenicity or ectopic pregnancy if emergency contraception fails and pregnancy ensues

Common Gynecologic Issues

TRACY A. BATTAGLIA, MD, MPH
MARIE ELLEN CAGGIANO
PHYLLIS L. CARR, MD
KAREN M. FREUND, MD, MPH
MARY GAUTHIER-DELAPLANE, MD
NEDA LAITEERAPONG
JANET F. McLAREN, MD
MARY ELLEN PAVONE, MD
HOPE A. RICCIOTTI, MD
MICHELE SINOPOLI, MD
TIFFANY JILL WERBIN, BSc, MA

16. Regulation of the Menstrual Cycle

Hypothalamic-Pituitary Axis
- The hypothalamus controls the pulsatile release of gonadotropin-releasing hormone
- The pituitary controls the pulsatile release of luteinizing hormone (LH) and follicle-stimulating hormone (FSH)
- The ovaries are involved in follicular development and cyclic secretion of estradiol, progesterone, and inhibin

Menstrual Cycle Phases
- **Follicular phase**
  - In response to withdrawal of estrogen and progesterone during the luteal phase of the prior menstrual cycle, the release of FSH from the pituitary results in the development of an ovarian follicle
  - The primordial follicle, in which the oocyte is surrounded by granulosa and theca cells, represents the earliest stage of follicular development
  - LH stimulates the theca cells to divide and produce androgens
  - FSH simulates the granulosa cells to produce the aromatase enzymes necessary to covert theca androgens to estrogens
  - The ovarian follicle produces estrogen, which enhances its own maturation by increasing the production of FSH and LH receptors in an autocrine fashion
  - The estradiol also induces endometrial proliferation, which prepares the uterus for implantation
  - The dominant follicle prevents the growth of other new follicles by inhibition feedback on FSH through estrogen, progesterone, and inhibin
  - Follicles destined for atresia have not captured enough FSH to complete maturation

- **Ovulation**
  - At mid-cycle, estradiol concentrations produced by the dominant follicle rise rapidly
  - When enough sustained estrogen is produced for 48 hours, the hypothalamic pituitary unit responds by secreting a surge of gonadotropins LH and FSH
  - There is an increase in LH pulse frequency and amplitude
  - The beginning of the LH surge precedes ovulation by approximately 35–44 hours
  - Ovulation occurs when the increase in LH levels cause the follicle to rupture and release the mature ovum

- **Luteal phase**
  - After ovulation, the follicle collapses and undergoes reorganization; the granulosa cells luteinize, developing receptors on their surface for cholesterol, which is a major precursor for the production of progesterone
  - Progesterone maintains the endometrial lining in preparation for receiving a fertilized ovum
  - If fertilization does not occur, the corpus luteum regresses and progesterone levels fall
  - The withdrawal of progesterone results in the endometrial lining sloughing off, causing menstruation
  - The lower levels of estrogen, progesterone, and inhibin induces the pituitary gland to increase gonadotropin secretion, and a new cycle of follicular recruitment begins

Two-cell system
- Theca interna cells produce androstenedione and testosterone in response to LH stimulation
- Granulosa cells, when stimulated by FSH, respond by increasing their ability to metabolize androgens to estrogens

Ovarian Regulatory Proteins
- Estradiol is secreted by the ovary and carried in the circulation to the pituitary gland, where it inhibits FSH secretions
- FSH stimulates the secretion of inhibin from ovarian granulosa cells; these proteins travel in the circulation to the pituitary gland where they markedly inhibit FSH secretion; the feedback inhibin on pituitary FSH secretion is critical to development of a single dominant follicle

Interconversion of Androgens and Estrogens
- All estrogen production is derived from androgens
- Androstenedione is converted to estrone by aromatase
- Testosterone is converted to estradiol by aromatase
- Aromatase activity is significant in the ovarian granulosa cell and the placenta; adipose tissue also contains aromatase

Menstruation
- During the follicular phase, the endometrium is in the proliferative phase and grows in response to estrogen
- During the luteal phase, the endometrium enters the secretory phase as it matures and is prepared to support implantation
- In the absence of fertilization, the decline in estrogen and progesterone levels cause the endometrium to slough, thereby initiating the menstrual phase

17. Premenstrual Syndrome

Etiology/Pathophysiology

- A constellation of physical and behavioral symptoms that repetitively occur during the second half of the menstrual cycle
- 80% of women suffer from symptoms of premenstrual syndrome (PMS)
- 5% of women are incapacitated by premenstrual dysphoric disorder, the most severe form of PMS
- Etiology is unknown
  - Genetic predisposition and sociocultural influences may play a role
  - PMS is cross-cultural and has been reported across ethnic groups and in different societies
  - Multiple studies have failed to show abnormal estradiol or progesterone levels in patients with PMS
- Hypotheses for the pathophysiology include dysfunction of CNS neurotransmitters (including the GABA and opiate systems and molecules involved in alterations of the adrenergic or the more studied serotonergic pathways), abnormal response to normal estrogen and progesterone level changes, and excess prostaglandin production

Differential Dx

- Mood disorders: Major depression, dysthymic disorder
- Anxiety disorder
- Hyperthyroidism
- Hypothyroidism
- Perimenopause
- Migraine
- Chronic fatigue syndrome
- Irritable bowel syndrome

Presentation

- A constellation of symptoms that occur only during the second half of the menstrual cycle
  - Extreme fatigue (90%)
  - Abdominal bloating (90%)
  - Mood lability (80%)
  - Marked increase in appetite or food preferences (70%)
  - Breast tenderness (50%)
  - Headache (50%)
  - Forgetfulness/difficulty concentrating (>50%)
  - Feeling sad, hopeless, or self-deprecating
  - Feeling tense, anxious, or "on-edge"
  - Persistent irritability, anger, and increased interpersonal conflicts

Diagnosis/Evaluation

- History of regular menstrual cycles
- Presence of symptoms characteristic of PMS and during the luteal phase of menstruation that impair the patient's socioeconomic functioning
- Patient must record symptoms prospectively for 2 months
  - A symptom-free interval that is clearly present during the follicular phase is required for a diagnosis of PMS
  - If there is no symptom-free interval during the follicular phase, the patient should be evaluated for a mood or anxiety disorder
- Absence of hormone or drug ingestion
- Chemistries, CBC, and serum TSH within normal limits

Treatment

- Continuous low-dose SSRIs have shown the most efficacy (e.g., fluoxetine, sertraline, anafranil)
- Alprazolam is indicated if SSRIs fail to improve symptoms
- Gonadotropin-releasing hormone agonists (e.g., Lupron) are used on patients who fail to respond to the above therapies
  - Therapy may be extended beyond 6 months with "add-back" therapy
  - Danazol is less preferred due to side effect profile
- NSAIDs or oral contraceptives may provide partial relief of physical symptoms
- Diuretics (e.g., thiazides, spironolactone) for severe edema

Prognosis/Complications

- Most women with PMS obtain significant relief with treatment
- The response rate for SSRIs is 60–75%
- In most women, PMS subsides at menopause
- Complications without treatment include depression and an increased incidence of suicide during the second half of the menstrual cycle

18. Abnormal Vaginal Bleeding

Etiology/Pathophysiology

- Defined as any irregular bleeding during the menstrual cycle
  - Menorrhagia, metrorrhagia, and polymenorrhea are associated with chronic anovulation, endometrial or cervical cancer, fibroids, endometrial hyperplasia, endometrial polyps, bleeding disorders, and complications of pregnancy
  - Hypomenorrhea is associated with hypogonadotropic hypogonadism (anorexics and athletes), atrophic endometrium, Asherman syndrome, oral contraceptive pills (OCPs), hormone replacement therapy (HRT), intrauterine adhesions, intrauterine trauma, and outlet obstructions (cervical stenosis or congenital abnormalities)
  - Oligomenorrhea is associated with pregnancy and disruptions of the pituitary-gonadal axis (e.g., premature ovarian failure)
- "Dysfunctional uterine bleeding" is a term that describes idiopathic heavy and/or irregular bleeding (commonly near menarche and menopause)

Differential Dx

- Anovulation
- Atrophic endometrium
- Pregnancy
- Premalignant lesions or malignancies (e.g., endometrial carcinoma or hyperplasia, cervical or vaginal cancer)
- Benign lesions (e.g., polyp, ovarian cysts, leiomyomata)
- Cervicitis, vaginitis, endometritis
- Trauma, foreign object
- Medical disease (e.g., liver, kidney, thyroid)
- Drugs (e.g., OCPs, HRT, anticoagulants)

Presentation

- Menorrhagia: Loss of >80 mL of blood in one menstrual cycle (1 pad/hr)
- Metrorrhagia: Bleeding between periods
- Hypomenorrhea: Unusually light menses
- Polymenorrhea: Frequent periods <21 days apart (usually caused by anovulation)
- Oligomenorrhea: Periods >35 days apart (frequently due to pregnancy)

Diagnosis/Evaluation

- Initial evaluation includes history and physical, pregnancy testing (serum β-hCG), hormonal tests, and Pap smear
  - History should evaluate timing and quantity of bleeding, menstrual history (e.g., menarche, recent periods, associated symptoms), and family history of bleeding disorders
  - Physical exam should rule out vaginal and cervical causes of bleeding and evaluate for uterine and adnexal masses
  - Hormonal tests include prolactin, TSH, LH, and FSH
  - Pap smear to screen for cervical cancer
- Further testing may be indicated based on clinical findings
  - Pelvic ultrasound to assess for polyps or fibroids
  - Hysterosalpingogram to assess for intrauterine defects
  - Sonohystogram to assess for polyps or submucosal fibroids
  - Endometrial biopsy (especially if age >35) to screen for endometrial hyperplasia and cancer
  - If unable to obtain endometrial biopsy, a hysteroscopy may be used to directly visualize the intrauterine cavity or D & C may be used to provide tissue for diagnosis

Treatment

- Medical treatment is effective in most cases
  - Oral contraceptive pills are often an effective first-line treatment for anovulatory bleeding, menorrhagia, metrorrhagia, and polymenorrhea
  - Progestin therapy can be used to treat anovulatory bleeding if estrogen is contraindicated (e.g., patients with endometrial hyperplasia)
  - Provera therapy for 10 days to treat menorrhagia
- Hysteroscopy may be used to remove fibroids and polyps
  - If hysteroscopy fails, proceed to endometrial ablation and resection of fibroids and polyps by laser, electrocautery, or heated roller
- D & C may be diagnostic and therapeutic for dysfunctional bleeding
- Hysterectomy is the definitive treatment for cases refractory to all other treatments

Prognosis/Complications

- Adolescents have an excellent prognosis; most outgrow the problem within 3–5 years of menarche
- Patients on oral contraceptives rarely have recurrent episodes
- For patients with abnormal bleeding related to systemic disease, prognosis depends on the underlying illness
  - Thyroid disorders have an excellent prognosis with correction of the underlying cause and/or hormone therapy
  - Successful therapy of PCOS is related to the amount of weight loss achieved
- Endometrial, cervical, or vaginal cancer depends on the stage of disease

19. Amenorrhea

Etiology/Pathophysiology

- Primary amenorrhea: Failure of the onset of menstruation by age 16
  - Etiologies include congenital abnormalities (e.g., imperforate hymen, uterine/vaginal agenesis), hormonal aberrations (e.g., androgen insensitivity, Savage syndrome), chromosomal abnormalities (e.g., Turner syndrome, Swyer syndrome), and hypothalamic-pituitary disorders (e.g., Kallmann syndrome, trauma)
- Secondary amenorrhea: Missed menses for 3 cycles or 6 months in a female who previously had normal menstruation
  - Etiologies include pregnancy, anatomic abnormalities (e.g., Asherman syndrome, cervical stenosis), ovarian dysfunction or premature ovarian failure, prolactinomas and hyperprolactinemia, and CNS/hypothalamic disorders (e.g., anorexia nervosa, excessive exercise, Sheehan syndrome)

Differential Dx

- Gonadal dysgenesis
- Chromosomal abnormality
- Vaginal atresia or agenesis
- Transverse vaginal septum
- Imperforate hymen
- Hypogonadotropism
- Hypopituitarism
- Pregnancy
- Anovulation
- Asherman syndrome
- Cervical stenosis
- Cushing's syndrome
- Pituitary tumor/infarct
- Thyroid disease

Presentation

- Primary amenorrhea: No menstruation by the age of 16
  - Imperforate hymen: Bulging bluish transparent membrane
  - Androgen insensitivity: 46, XY genotype, blind vaginal pouch with absence of uterus and ovaries
- Secondary amenorrhea: Missed menses for 3 cycles or 6 months in a female with previously normal cycles
  - Ovarian dysfunction/failure: Hot flashes, mood swings, vaginal dryness, dyspareunia, skin thinning
  - Prolactinoma/hyperprolactinemia: Headache, diplopia, gynecomastia, galactorrhea, and virilization
  - Sheehan syndrome: Failure to lactate, fatigue, and failure to resume menstruation

Diagnosis/Evaluation

- Test for pregnancy and assess for patency of vagina
- TSH and prolactin levels
- Progestin challenge test to assess for the presence of estrogen and an adequate outflow tract
- FSH and LH levels
  - Low FSH and LH suggest hypothalamic/pituitary disorder
  - High FSH and LH suggest ovarian failure
- Absence of withdrawal bleeding from estrogen and progesterone with normal hormone levels may indicate an outflow tract disorder (e.g., Asherman syndrome, cervical stenosis)
- If uterus and/or breasts are absent: Karyotype analysis, followed by testosterone and serum FSH levels
  - Breasts absent/uterus present: FSH >40 mIU/mL = hypergonadotropic hypogonadism; FSH <40 mIU/mL = hypogonadotropic hypogonadism
  - Uterus absent/breasts present: Karyotype differentiates between Müllerian agenesis and testicular feminization
  - Absent uterus and breasts: karyotype is usually 46, XY

Treatment

- Ovarian dysfunction: Oral contraceptive pills
- Ovarian failure: Hormone replacement therapy
- Asherman syndrome: Hysteroscopic lysis of adhesions followed by hormone therapy
- Pituitary microadenoma/hyperprolactinemia: Excision or medical treatment with bromocriptine
- Pituitary macroadenoma: Surgical resection
- Hypothalamic dysfunction: Correct the underlying cause and induce ovulation with gonadotropins
- Congenital abnormalities: Plastic surgery to allow outflow of menses or to create a functional vagina
- Androgen insensitivity: Testes should be surgically excised because of risk of testicular cancer

Prognosis/Complications

- Overall the prognosis is good, depending on the etiology; in most cases, symptoms and conditions related to amenorrhea are reversible and treatable
- If amenorrhea is secondary, the possibility is good for correcting the amenorrhea, through medication, lifestyle change, or surgery
- Chromosomal abnormalities are unlikely to be corrected by any intervention
- Complications include psychological distress or crisis and failure of proper bone growth and/or osteoporosis

20. Dysmenorrhea & Pelvic Pain

Etiology/Pathophysiology

- Dysmenorrhea: Pain and cramping during menstruation that interferes with normal function; affects 50% of women; 1% become incapacitated for 1–3 days
  - Primary dysmenorrhea (75% of cases): Menstrual pain in the absence of underlying pelvic disease that occurs with ovulatory menstrual cycles; may be related to prostaglandins F_{2a} or E_2 released from the endometrium during menstruation or higher tissue levels of prostaglandins
  - Secondary dysmenorrhea (25% of cases): Menstrual pain due to pelvic disease, including endometriosis/adenomyosis (80%), pelvic adhesions (20%), chronic PID, uterine leiomyomata, cervical stenosis
- Pelvic pain: Pain localized below the level of the umbilicus that interferes with normal function
  - May be of gynecologic, gastrointestinal, urinary, musculoskeletal, or psychological etiology
  - Chronic pelvic pain affects 15% of women ages 18–50
  - 25% of these women spend a day in bed each month due to their pain
  - 35% of laparoscopies are performed for chronic pelvic pain

Differential Dx

- Endometriosis/adeno-myosis
- Leiomyoma
- PID
- Ectopic pregnancy
- Ovarian/adnexal torsion
- Hemorrhagic cyst
- Ruptured TOA
- Appendicitis
- Diverticulitis
- IBS
- Abdominal hernia
- Nephrolithiasis
- Chronic UTI
- Constipation
- Fibromyalgia
- Cancer

Presentation

- Primary dysmenorrhea: Cramping and lower abdominal discomfort most severe at onset of menses and lasting 12–72 hours; associated symptoms include nausea, vomiting, diarrhea, and headache; usually begins in adolescence
- Secondary dysmenorrhea: Pain may be similar to menstrual cramps but usually begins earlier in the menstrual cycle and lasts longer than the menses; associated symptoms vary depending on the pathology; later age of onset (after age 25–30)
- Pelvic pain: Discomfort or pain localized to below the umbilicus; associated symptoms vary depending on the pathology

Diagnosis/Evaluation

- Obtain a complete menstrual and gynecologic history, history of symptoms, past medical history, psychosocial history, and medication and dietary history
- Abdominal exam should assess for surgical scars, hernias, masses, tenderness, rigidity, rebound tenderness, or guarding
- Pelvic exam should evaluate for signs of infection (including vaginal wet mount and testing for chlamydia and gonorrhea if warranted); uterosacral ligament abnormalities; cervical stenosis, motion tenderness, or lateral displacement of the cervix; and uterine or adnexal tenderness
- Rectal exam to rule out masses and assess for point tenderness
- Lab tests may include β-hCG, Pap smear, urinalysis, and CBC
- Pelvic and vaginal ultrasound are used to assess for lower abdominal and pelvic pathology (e.g., ovarian/adnexal torsion, nephrolithiasis, appendicitis, hemorrhagic cysts, fibroids)
- Hysteroscopy or hysterosalpingogram may be indicated
- Operative laparoscopy may be necessary to diagnose and remove endometriosis, adhesions, ovarian cysts, fibroids, appendicitis, and other gastrointestinal or renal pathologies

Treatment

- Primary dysmenorrhea
  - Nonpharmacologic therapies include rest, use of heating pad on the lower abdomen or back, and lifestyle changes (e.g., regular exercise, smoking cessation, decrease in alcohol and caffeine consumption, weight reduction)
  - Pharmacologic therapies include NSAIDs (start 1 day before expected onset of symptoms and continue through menses) and oral contraceptives (first-line if contraception is desired and no contraindications)
- Secondary dysmenorrhea: NSAIDs, OCPs, GnRH agonists (leuprolide or nafarelin), progestin therapy, doxycycline (empiric treatment for some causes of PID), and operative laparoscopy or open surgery
- Pelvic pain: Empiric treatment similar to dysmenorrhea
  - Surgical interventions include cystoscopy or laparoscopic resection of pathology
  - Presacral neurectomy may be indicated for resistant chronic pelvic pain

Prognosis/Complications

- Primary dysmenorrhea: Symptoms usually become less painful with age
  - A pregnancy carried to viability will usually decrease symptoms
  - After 1 year of OCP use, most patients experience a reduction of symptoms, even if OCPs are discontinued
- Secondary dysmenorrhea: Prognosis is often good if appropriately diagnosed and treated
  - Some etiologies may result in infertility if left untreated
- Pelvic pain: Prognosis is often good if appropriately diagnosed and treated
  - True emergencies (e.g., ruptured tubal pregnancy, PID, appendicitis) may be life threatening if untreated

21. Functional Ovarian Cysts

Etiology/Pathophysiology

- 75% of ovarian masses in women of reproductive age are functional cysts; 25% are neoplasms
- Functional cysts result from the normal physiologic action of the ovary
- Functional cysts include follicular, corpus luteum, and theca lutein cysts
    - Follicular cysts arise after failure of the follicle to rupture during maturation; most resolve spontaneously within 4–6 weeks
    - Corpus lutein cysts occur during the luteal phase (second half) of the menstrual cycle, when the corpus luteum becomes enlarged (>3 cm), hemorrhagic, or fails to regress after 14 days
    - Theca lutein cysts are numerous, bilateral luteinized follicle cysts (immature ovarian follicles), which are due to stimulation by abnormally high β-hCG levels (e.g., due to a molar pregnancy, choriocarcinoma, or clomiphene therapy)

Differential Dx

- Ovarian neoplasms
- Ectopic pregnancy
- Hydrosalpinx
- Tubo-ovarian abscess
- Paraovarian cyst
- Peritoneal inclusion cyst
- Diverticular or appendiceal abscess
- Pelvic inflammatory disease
- Inflammatory bowel disease
- Fallopian tube cancer

Presentation

- Cysts generally present as asymptomatic adnexal masses that are palpated during pelvic exam
- Large follicular cysts may cause aching pelvic pain, dyspareunia, or ovarian torsion; symptoms often develop during mid-cycle
- Corpus lutein cysts may cause pelvic pain (usually in the second half of the menstrual cycle), amenorrhea, or delayed menses
- Theca lutein cysts are bilateral and numerous, and may be secondary to clomiphene therapy for ovulation induction or the stimulatory effects of molar pregnancy and choriocarcinoma

Diagnosis/Evaluation

- Physical examination, including pelvic and rectovaginal examination
- β-hCG measurement to evaluate for pregnancy
- CBC if there is evidence of intraperitoneal bleeding
- Ultrasound is the primary diagnostic tool for the evaluation of adnexal masses/ovarian cysts
    - The size, structure, and general appearance of the cysts will guide in the diagnosis; however, hemorrhage or clot formation around the cyst may obscure the appearance
    - Functional cysts typically appear as simple, unilocular cysts without papillary vegetations or thickened walls
- In premenopausal women, cysts are usually observed for 6 weeks; if they resolve, a diagnosis of a functional cyst is made
- In postmenopausal or premenarcheal patients, ovarian cysts are likely to be neoplasms and should be investigated surgically; a CA-125 level may be obtained in postmenopausal women to aid in management

Treatment

- In premenopausal women, cysts are usually followed for 4–6 weeks; if they resolve, a diagnosis of a functional cyst is made and no further treatment is needed
- In postmenopausal women, surgical removal is recommended due to the higher incidence of malignancy
- In premenarcheal women, ovarian cysts are unlikely to be functional; surgical exploration is usually required
- Cysts that do not resolve require surgical exploration (laparotomy or laparoscopy) so that a histologic diagnosis may be made and to prevent ovarian torsion
- Multilocular ovarian cysts diagnosed by ultrasound (with or without solid parts) should be surgically removed, especially in postmenopausal women; the more complex the tumor, the higher the risk of malignancy
- Oral contraceptives may be used to diminish ovarian activity and possibly decrease the incidence of recurrent ovarian cysts

Prognosis/Complications

- Functional ovarian cysts may cause ovarian torsion
- Bleeding from a hemorrhagic corpus luteum can result in acute abdominal pain or cystic rupture
- Approximately 90% of simple ovarian cysts that are followed more than 9 weeks resolve

22. Polycystic Ovarian Syndrome

Etiology/Pathophysiology

- Previously known as Stein-Leventhal syndrome
- A syndrome of androgen excess, possibly due to excess LH stimulation of the ovaries
- Presents with the classic clinical triad of hirsutism, anovulation, and obesity
- Polycystic ovaries each contain at least eight small (2–8 mm) follicles
- Chronic oligo- or anovulation occurs due to functional ovarian hyperandrogenism (80%) and/or functional adrenal hyperandrogenism (50%)
- Etiology is unknown; proposed theories include excess of trophic hormones (LH or ACTH) amplified by disturbances in intrinsic (inhibin and/or follisatin) or extrinsic (insulin or insulin-like growth factor) regulatory peptides; dysregulation of steroidogenesis (presence of an intrinsic ovarian genetic disorder that requires a "second hit" to precipitate the syndrome)

Differential Dx

- CAH
- Hyperprolactinemia
- Cushing syndrome
- Acromegaly
- Ovarian tumors (e.g., Sertoli-Leydig cell tumors)
- Ovarian steroidogenic block (e.g., aromatase deficiency)
- Adrenal tumors
- Drugs (e.g., danazol, OCPs with androgenic progestins)
- Hyperthecosis
- Severe insulin resistance syndromes

Presentation

- Menstrual irregularity: Oligo- or anovulation, amenorrhea, irregular bleeding
- Evidence of hyperandrogenism: Hirsutism, acne, or alopecia
- Obesity
- Diabetes mellitus
- Infertility
- Premature pubarche and precocious puberty
- Acanthosis nigricans (insulin resistance)

Diagnosis/Evaluation

- Diagnosis depends on clinical and/or biochemical evidence of hyperandrogenism
- Ultrasound may reveal polycystic ovaries (80–100%); however, the isolated finding of polycystic ovaries (without hyperandrogenism) is very common and does not constitute disease
- Laboratory studies
  - Elevated LH/FSH ratio >3 (suggestive but not diagnostic)
  - Exaggerated pulsatile LH levels
  - Elevated androgens (androstenedione and testosterone)
  - Low serum steroidal hormone-binding globulin (SHBG), resulting in elevated free testosterone levels
  - Normal prolactin level
  - Elevated Hb_{A1c} and random blood glucose
  - Consider checking insulin level to determine the need for metformin

Treatment

- Administer oral contraceptives to regulate the menstrual cycle and for endometrial protection
- Improve insulin resistance via weight loss and insulin sensitizing drugs (e.g., metformin)
  - Ensure adequate contraception in patients using metformin
- Treat hirsutism via hair removal by shaving, depilatories, electrolysis, or laser treatment; oral contraceptives with or without an anti-androgen (e.g., spironolactone)
- In patients who desire pregnancy, initial choices include clomiphene or metformin to induce ovulation
  - Persistent cases may be treated with assisted reproductive techonologies (e.g., invitro fertilization)
  - If pregnancy is achieved, there is a high incidence of gestational diabetes

Prognosis/Complications

- This syndrome is not curable; however, with proper diagnosis and treatment, including weight loss and diet, most symptoms can be adequately controlled or eliminated
- In most women, pregnancy can be achieved with appropriate medical interventions
- Associated complications include
  - Sterility
  - Diabetes (glucose levels should be checked regularly)
  - Negative self-image
  - Increased risk of endometrial hyperplasia and endometrial cancer due to oligo-ovulation
  - Risk of cardiac disease due to elevated cholesterol and triglycerides

23. Hirsutism & Virilization

Etiology/Pathophysiology

- Hirsutism is an increase in androgen-dependent terminal hair (stiff, thick, pigmented hair) in a *male distribution* on the face, back, chest, and abdomen
  - Occurs in response to excess androgens—in the majority of cases, excessive androgen production is secondary to anovulation
  - Differentiate from hypertrichosis, which refers to diffusely increased non-androgen-dependent total body hair and is reversible
  - One-third of women ages 14–45 have excessive upper lip hair
  - 6–9% have unwanted chin/sideburn hair
- Virilization is the development of a constellation of male features, including hirsutism, deepening voice, frontal balding, clitoromegaly, and increased musculature
  - Etiology is primarily adrenal or ovarian disorders, including polycystic ovarian syndrome, ovarian tumors, adrenal tumors, congenital adrenal hyperplasia, and Cushing syndrome

Differential Dx

- Hypertrichosis
  - Drugs (e.g., steroids, phenytoin, diazoxide, cyclosporine)
  - Pathologic states (e.g., hypothyroidism, anorexia)
- Endogenous androgen overproduction
  - Tumors (pituitary, adrenal, ovarian)
  - Non-tumors (e.g., congenital adrenal hyperplasia, Cushing syndrome)
  - Androgenized ovary syndrome
- Idiopathic hirsutism

Presentation

- Male body hair distribution
  - Face: Mustache, beard, sideburns
  - Body: Chest, circumareolar, linea alba, abdominal trigone, inner thighs
- Breast atrophy
- Frontal balding
- Deepening voice
- Clitoromegaly
- Increased musculature or absence of female contours
- Acanthosis nigricans (velvety, thickened hyperpigmented skin) in the axilla and back of neck

Diagnosis/Evaluation

- History should include time course of symptoms (progressive worsening, late age of onset, or abrupt onset suggest a tumor)
- Laboratory studies
  - Testosterone level of 50–150 ng/dL suggests an endocrine disorder; levels >200 ng/dL require imaging studies
  - LH/FSH ratio >3 suggests polycystic ovarian syndrome
  - DHEAS level should be measured if progressive symptoms, irregular menstrual cycles, or any signs of virilization (>700 μg/dL suggests adrenal hyperplasia or tumor)
  - 17-hydroxyprogesterone <300 ng/dL or suppressible rules out adrenal hyperplasia
  - Prolactin and TSH should be measured if menstrual cycles are irregular
- Imaging studies are indicated if blood studies suggest a tumor
  - Abdominal CT scan to rule out an adrenal tumor
  - Pelvic ultrasound or CT scan to rule out an ovarian tumor
- Endometrial biopsy to evaluate for endometrial hyperplasia if periods are irregular and there is concern for PCOS

Treatment

- Treat the underlying cause to prevent growth of terminal hair (in most cases, the cause is hyperandrogenism secondary to anovulation)
  - Combination low-dose estrogen and non-androgenic progestin OCPs will inhibit adrenal and ovarian androgen production, stimulate SHBG production by the liver, and diminish terminal hair growth
  - Spironolactone (anti-androgen therapy) blocks the binding of testosterone to its receptors
- Remove terminal hair by waxing, depilatories, electrolysis, or laser treatment
- GnRH agonist (e.g., luprolide) in combination with an OCP or estrogen may be used if other therapies fail
- All currently available medications for hirsutism must be stopped if pregnancy is desired
- Dexamethasone will reduce virilization secondary to adrenal hyperplasia

Prognosis/Complications

- Hair removal and oral contraceptive use generally provide good results
- Idiopathic hirsutism and PCOS are usually not reversible; however, if untreated, a gradual increase in terminal hair growth may occur with age
- There is no cure for virilization due to adrenal hyperplasia; however, it can usually be controlled with ongoing glucocorticoid treatment
- Patients with virilization due to a cancerous tumor have a better prognosis with early diagnosis and treatment

24. Endometriosis & Adenomyosis

Etiology/Pathophysiology

- Endometriosis is the presence of endometrial tissue outside the endometrial cavity (most often on the ovary or pelvic peritoneum)
  - Etiology is unknown; hypotheses include retrograde menstruation, coelomic metaplasia, and hematogenous or lymphatic spread
  - 10–15% occurrence rate; less often in black women
  - Nearly 10% genetic predisposition
  - Occurs in reproductive-aged women; 20% have chronic pelvic pain; 30–40% have infertility
  - Accounts for 50% of cases of chronic pelvic pain or dysmenorrhea in adolescents
- Adenomyosis is a type of endometriosis in which endometrial tissue is found within the myometrium (endometriosis interna), resulting in hypertrophy and hyperplasia
  - 15% occurrence rate
  - Generally occurs in parous women in their late 30–40s
  - 15% have associated endometriosis
  - 50–60% have associated fibroids

Differential Dx

- Dysmenorrhea
- Pelvic inflammatory disease
- Interstitial cystitis
- Acute salpingitis
- Fibroids
- Adhesions
- Hemorrhagic corpus luteum
- Ovarian neoplasms

Presentation

- Endometriosis symptoms may not correlate with the extent of disease
  - Dysmenorrhea
  - Dyspareunia
  - Infertility
  - Abnormal bleeding
  - Cyclic pelvic pain
  - Pre- and postmenstrual spotting
  - Ovulatory pain
  - Mid-cycle bleeding
- Adenomyosis
  - Asymptomatic in 20%
  - Dysmenorrhea in 30%
  - Menorrhagia in 50%
  - Globally enlarged uterus

Diagnosis/Evaluation

- Endometriosis
  - Findings on bimanual exam may include tenderness when palpating the posterior fornix; uterosacral nodularity; fixed or retroverted uterus; or tender, enlarged adnexal masses
  - Direct visualization via laparoscopy or laparotomy and biopsy (may show rust-colored to dark brown "powder burns"; raised, purple-blue "mulberry" lesions; or "chocolate" ovarian cysts)
  - Mild to moderate elevation of serum CA-125 (not specific) correlates best with advanced disease
- Adenomyosis
  - Bimanual exam reveals a soft, symmetrically enlarged uterus
  - Biopsy of myometrium via operative hysteroscopy or laparoscopy
  - MRI
  - Often found incidentally on pathologic examination of hysterectomy specimens

Treatment

- Endometriosis
  - NSAIDs
  - Medical induction of "pseudopregnancy" with oral contraceptive pills or progestins
  - Medical induction of "pseudomenopause" with gonadotropin-releasing hormone agonists with or without oral contraceptives or danazol sulfate
  - Conservative surgical treatment may include laser ablation or electrocauterization of implants and adhesions
  - Definitive surgical treatment is by total abdominal hysterectomy with bilateral salpingo-oopherectomy (TAH–BSO), lysis of adhesions, and removal of endometriosis lesions
- Adenomyosis
  - Conservative treatment with NSAIDs for mild cases
  - Definitive treatment is hysterectomy

Prognosis/Complications

- Medical treatment is generally only of temporary relief
- The success of conservative surgical treatment depends on the extent of disease
  - 75% post-surgery pregnancy rates for mild disease
  - 50–60% post-surgery pregnancy rates for moderate disease
  - 30–40% post-surgery pregnancy rates for severe disease
- Definitive surgical treatment is reserved for cases in which childbearing is complete or for refractory cases

25. Fibroids

Etiology/Pathophysiology

- Uterine leiomyomas, also known as fibroids, are benign tumors composed of uterine smooth muscle cells and extracellular matrix
- Fibroids are clinically apparent in 20–25% of women of reproductive age
- Fibroids are described by their location:
    - Submucosal: Underlie and distort the endometrial layer
    - Intramural: Lie within the uterine muscular wall
    - Subserosal: Underlie the uterine serosa and can be pedunculated
- The growth pattern of fibroids follows the reproductive life cycle: They are stimulated by estrogen and progesterone and regress after menopause
- The pathophysiology of fibroid formation is not well understood; they arise from smooth muscle cells of the myometrium; sarcomatous transformation is thought *not* to occur
- Women of color have a two- to three-fold greater incidence of fibroid formation for unknown reasons
- Some evidence suggests that higher parity, oral contraceptive use, and smoking decrease the risk of fibroid formation

Differential Dx

- Leiomyosarcoma
- Adenomyoma
- Gravid uterus
- Adnexal mass

Presentation

- 20–50% of women with fibroids have symptoms; many are asymptomatic
- Uterine bleeding: Prolonged or heavy menstrual flow (menorrhagia) is most common with submucosal fibroids; may lead to anemia
- Pelvic pressure and pain: Bladder compression may lead to increased urinary frequency; compression of the colon may lead to constipation; dyspareunia may result from pressure on cervix and vagina
- Pregnancy: Distortion of uterine cavity may lead to miscarriage; placental implantation over a fibroid may lead to poor fetal blood supply or placental abruption; associated with premature labor and malposition

Diagnosis/Evaluation

- The diagnosis of fibroids is usually by bimanual examination; the uterus is enlarged, irregular, and may be palpated abdominally
- Fibroid size is described by menstrual weeks as in pregnancy
- Physical findings can be confirmed by imaging
    - Ultrasound is often used to visualize fibroids and is most sensitive for finding tumors in smaller uteri
    - MRI can best differentiate between fibroids, adenomyomas, and leiomyosarcomas
    - Imaging is also used to delineate the location of fibroids, as when planning for surgical removal
    - Hysterosalpingogram, sonohysterogram, or hysteroscopy may be used to evaluate the shape of the endometrial cavity, most often in a fertility evaluation

Treatment

- Treatment is indicated for large or symptomatic fibroids
- Surgical therapy: Fibroids are the most common indication for hysterectomy; reserved for women who are not interested in childbearing; myomectomy may be performed to preserve childbearing potential; depending upon fibroid size/location, myomectomy can be done abdominally, laparoscopically, or hysteroscopically
- Medical therapy: Treatment with GnRH analogs induces amenorrhea, allowing anemic women to increase hemoglobin concentrations; cessation of therapy results in rapid regrowth of leiomyomas to pretreatment volume; thus, primarily useful as a presurgical treatment but not as a long-term treatment option; combinations of GnRH agonists and low dosages of estrogen ("add-back") are used to extend the maximal duration of therapy
- Uterine artery embolization is effective for fibroid regression and symptomatic relief; reserved for those patients who are finished with childbearing

Prognosis/Complications

- Fibroids tend to regress following menopause; therefore, asymptomatic fibroids can be managed expectantly; women with fibroids tend to develop new tumors as long as they are exposed to reproductive hormones
- Myomectomy diminishes menorrhagia in 80% of patients; fibroids can recur, with ultrasonographic evidence of recurrence in 25–50% of patients; up to 10% require a second major operative procedure; myomectomy results in an increased risk of uterine rupture in future labor
- Pressure of the myomatous uterus on the ureters resulting in hydronephrosis is a rare indication for surgical intervention

26. Breast Mass Evaluation

Etiology/Pathophysiology

- A palpable breast mass is defined as a dominant mass if it is three-dimensional, distinct from surrounding tissue, asymmetrical to the other breast, and persists through a menstrual cycle
- Indirect evidence supports the effectiveness of the clinical breast exam: Sensitivity range is 40–69%; specificity range is 86–99%; positive predictive value range is 4–50%
- 4% of abnormal exams are subsequently diagnosed with cancer
- The age-specific incidence of benign disorders drops after menopause, but benign disorders are still more frequent than cancer up to age 75
- The two most common benign breast masses are cysts and fibroadenomas
  - Gross cystic disease is found in approximately 7% of adult women in the U.S.; most frequent in the fourth decade and in perimenopause; arise from dilatation or obstruction of the collecting ducts
  - Fibroadenomas are the most frequent benign tumor in young women; median age at diagnosis is 30 years; arise from proliferation of periductal stromal connective tissue within the lobules of the breast; growth is stimulated by exogenous estrogen, progesterone, lactation, and pregnancy

Differential Dx

- Nonproliferative
  - Cyst (simple vs complex)
  - Fibroadenoma
  - Physiologic nodularity
  - Ductal ectasia
  - Reactive lymph node
  - Lipoma
  - Sebaceous gland/cyst
- Proliferative disease without atypia
- Atypical hyperplasia
- Breast cancer

Presentation

- Breast tenderness or pain
- Normal physiologic nodularity (often incorrectly called fibrocystic disease) can be difficult to distinguish from a discrete mass (less likely to have clear borders, often cordlike, and often changes with menstrual cycle)
- Nipple discharge is rarely associated with a mass; bloody discharge is usually benign (95%), but requires evaluation

Diagnosis/Evaluation

- Collect historical information to establish baseline risk, including age, menstrual status, parity, family history, previous biopsy results, and exogenous hormone use
- Clinical breast examination should document approximate size, site, mobility, and texture, as well as associated skin retraction, erythema, or adenopathy
  - Benign features include smooth, well-demarcated, and mobile lesions
  - Malignant features include hard, irregular, and fixed lesions; bloody nipple discharge; skin dimpling; and nipple retraction
- Further diagnostic evaluation dependent on age
  - Under age 35: Ultrasound or fine needle aspiration indicated to determine whether lesion is cystic or solid
  - Over age 35: Diagnostic mammography should be done first; if lesion is benign-appearing or not seen on mammogram, then ultrasound is indicated to determine if cystic or solid

Treatment

- Cystic masses may be treated by observation with repeat clinical breast exam in 3–6 months or may be aspirated by a therapeutic fine needle aspiration in the office or a core needle biopsy under ultrasound guidance
  - Aspiration is indicated for complex cysts, simple cysts in postmenopausal woman, or symptomatic cysts (pain or anxiety)
  - Send fluid to cytology if bloody or complex
- All solid masses require tissue diagnosis
  - Fine needle aspiration biopsy OR
  - Core needle biopsy under ultrasound guidance OR
  - Excisional biopsy; required when clinically suspicious (hard, fixed, >1.5 cm), high risk (e.g., positive family history for breast cancer), or patient preference

Prognosis/Complications

- Cystic masses require follow up 4–6 weeks after aspiration to ensure no re-accumulation and every 6 months thereafter
  - Biopsy if re-accumulation occurs
- Solid masses require a tissue diagnosis
  - If fibroadenoma and <1 cm, follow clinically every 6 months
  - Despite normal breast tissue findings of a dominant mass by fine needle aspiration or core needle biopsy, an enlarging dominant mass requires surgical excision
- Frequent follow up (every 3–6 months) is warranted if an examination is particularly difficult in order to maintain familiarity and confirm stability

27. Galactorrhea

Etiology/Pathophysiology

- Galactorrhea is defined as inappropriate lactation (i.e., not associated with prior delivery of an infant)
- The female breast is primed by estrogen, progesterone, growth hormone, insulin, thyroid hormone, and glucocorticoids, which aid in the development of the ductal system, lobules, and secretory aspects of the alveoli; high levels of estrogen and progesterone inhibit lactation; the drop in these hormones after delivery, with an elevated prolactin level, facilitate lactation
- Galactorrhea may be due to abnormal hypothalamic inhibition, increased production of prolactin or any disease process that interferes with the connection between hypothalamus and pituitary
- The presence of galactorrhea usually indicates an underlying endocrinopathy; however, true galactorrhea must be differentiated from other breast secretions (e.g., the presence of a bloody or serous discharge can be associated with breast disease, including malignancy)
- Up to 20% of healthy women who have been pregnant in the past may have milky discharge at times, especially following nipple stimulation; however, nulliparous women rarely have "normal" discharge so require an endocrine workup

Differential Dx

- Idiopathic
- Drugs (phenothiazines, methyldopa, TCAs, estrogen)
- Pituitary adenoma
- Pituitary stalk resection
- Hypothyroidism (TRH stimulates prolactin)
- Chest wall stimulation (trauma, suck reflex)
- CNS disease (tumors, trauma, sarcoidosis, infections)
- Hydatidiform mole
- Choriocarcinoma
- Bronchogenic carcinoma

Presentation

- In true galactorrhea, the breast secretion is white and contains all the constituents of normal human milk
- Secretions issue from multiple ducts and usually occur in both breasts
- There should be no associated breast mass or breast pain; these symptoms increase suspicion of breast disease
- Women with prolactin-secreting pituitary adenomas may present with amenorrhea and infertility, as prolactin interferes with normal release of FSH and LH
- Headache, galactorrhea, amenorrhea, defects in peripheral vision, hirsutism, acne, hypogonadism, decreased libido, infertility, and bone density abnormalities may be present

Diagnosis/Evaluation

- Thorough history and physical examination, including menstrual history and medications
- Prolactin drawn immediately after breast exam, thyroid function, hCG (to rule out pregnancy)
- Hyperprolactinemia levels (note that levels may be elevated transiently and therefore not detected with a single lab draw)
- The higher the prolactin level, the more likely a pituitary tumor
- Mammography is not indicated unless physical exam is suggestive of brain pathology
- MRI/CT scan are used to evaluate the CNS for pathology (MRI with gadolinium enhancement for pituitary adenomas)
    - Any patient with a mass >1 cm should have a neurologic evaluation, including visual field testing
- Idiopathic galactorrhea is a diagnosis of exclusion

Treatment

- Drug-induced galactorrhea resolves when the medication is discontinued
- Dopaminergic agents such as bromocriptine suppress prolactin production and are used to treat prolactin-producing pituitary adenomas. These drugs may even be helpful in cases of idiopathic galactorrhea; orthostatic hypertension is a common side effect of bromocriptine therapy; patient education is critical to allow continuation of the drug
- Patients with physiologic galactorrhea (normal prolactin levels) should be reassured; they can be advised to avoid excessive breast stimulation, including repeated self-examinations or excessive nipple manipulation during sexual activity
- Treatment of the underlying disease process is necessary in hypothyroidism, CNS disease, and hormone-producing carcinomas

Prognosis/Complications

- Many patients initially diagnosed with idiopathic galactorrhea develop a detectable pituitary adenoma
- In 90% of patients with prolactinomas, bromocriptine results in shrinkage of the tumor and prolactin levels decrease. Nonresponders to medication (persistent hyperprolactinema, visual field deficits) at risk for osteoporosis; lower gonadotropin and estrogen levels decrease bone density; surgery and/or radiation may be useful
- Women with prolactinomas who become pregnant may experience tumor growth during pregnancy. Bromocriptine is not licensed for use during pregnancy and 5–15% of women will become symptomatic. Resolution usually occurs with delivery and resumption of therapy

28. Vulvovaginitis

Etiology/Pathophysiology

- Vulvovaginitis is an inflammation and irritation of the vagina and/or vulva
- Extremely common (over 10 million office visits per year)
- Bacterial vaginosis (BV) is the most common cause of abnormal vaginal discharge in women of childbearing age
  - Characterized by a change in normal vaginal flora: Decreased H_2O_2-producing lactobacilli and increase in other species, including *Gardnerella vaginalis*, *Mycoplasma hominis*, and gram-negative anaerobes
  - Risk factors include multiple sexual partners, new partner(s), and douching
  - Though infection rates are higher in sexually active populations, BV is *not* an STD
- Vulvovaginal candidiasis (VVC) caused by yeast, usually *Candida albicans*
  - Not an STD; most cases are sporadic
  - Risk factors for infection and recurrence include antibiotic use, OCP use, uncontrolled diabetes, and immunocompromise
- Trichomoniasis is sexually transmitted; caused by the protozoan *Trichomonas vaginalis*
- Atrophic vaginitis is characterized by thinning of the vaginal epithelium caused by reduced estrogen levels, most often associated with menopause

Differential Dx

- Normal vaginal discharge
- Vaginal infections (e.g., bacterial vaginosis, candidiasis, trichomoniasis)
- Cervicitis (chlamydia, gonorrhea)
- Herpes infections (particularly if fissures are present)
- Atrophic vaginitis
- Allergic, chemical, or mechanical irritation

Presentation

- Symptomatic BV presents with increased discharge, a "fishy odor," and few or no irritative symptoms
- VVC presents with irritation, pruritis, soreness, dysuria, and dyspareunia;
  - Discharge is white and thick ("cottage cheese" like)
- Trichomoniasis may be asymptomatic or result in severe inflammation
  - Discharge is yellow-green and malodorous
  - Punctate hemorrhages on the cervix give a classic "strawberry" appearance in 20% of women
- Atrophic vaginitis presents in post-menopausal women with spotty bleeding, post-coital bleeding, and dyspareunia

Diagnosis/Evaluation

- BV diagnosis requires three of four positive criteria (90% sensitivity)
  - Homogeneous grey-white discharge
  - pH >4.5
  - Positive "whiff test" for amine odor
  - Presence of clue cells on saline prep
  - Gram stain may also be used to make a diagnosis, and actually has a higher sensitivity (95%)
- VVC requires culture for *Candida* for definitive diagnosis
  - Normal pH (<4.5)
  - Pseudohyphae on 10% KOH prep may be seen in 60% of cases
- Trichomoniasis requires culture for *T. vaginalis* for definitive diagnosis
  - Motile protozoa are seen on saline prep in 70% of cases
  - pH is normal or elevated
- Atrophic vaginitis is a clinical diagnosis: Mucosa is visibly thinned, dry, and erythematous

Treatment

- BV: Symptomatic women should be treated with oral metronidazole (single dose or 7-day course) or vaginal metronidazole gel (5 days)
  - Clindamycin is also effective (vaginal cream for 10 days or orally for 5 days)
  - Pregnant women should be treated with metronidazole in a single dose, regardless of symptoms, as BV has been associated with adverse pregnancy outcomes
- VVC: Over-the-counter topical antifungals (85–90% effective) or a single dose of oral fluconazole
  - Terconazole is indicated for recurrent candidiasis (to cover *C. glabrata* and *C. tropicalis*)
- Trichomoniasis: Oral metronidazole (single dose or 7-day course)
  - Partners should be treated as well
  - Pregnant women require single dose therapy
- Atrophic vaginitis: Topical estrogen creams (2–3x/week)

Prognosis/Complications

- 30% of patients who are treated successfully for BV will have a recurrence within 3 months; however, suppressive therapy has not been shown to be useful
- 5% of patients will experience recurrent VVC; maintenance therapy (6 months) with oral antifungals may eradicate the infection in these cases
- There is an increasing incidence of metronidazole-resistant *Trichomonas*; treat with higher doses of metronidazole or concurrent topical and oral therapy
- Trichomoniasis during pregnancy has been associated with preterm labor and premature rupture of membranes (PROM)

29. Vulvar Disease

Etiology/Pathophysiology

- The most common causes of vulvar irritation are reactions to topical agents, including creams, soaps, talcs, or irritating synthetic fabrics in clothing
- Infections causing vulvar pathology include viruses (e.g., HPV, HSV, zoster, molluscum), parasites (e.g., pubic lice, scabies, pinworm), and mycotic infections (e.g., tinea, *Candida*), which cause severe vulvar dermatitis
- Vulvar dystrophies are benign disorders that result in atrophic and hypertrophic lesions; these include lichen sclerosus, squamous cell hyperplasia, lichen simplex chronicus, and lichen planus
  - Lichen sclerosus is the most common and is thought to be autoimmune
  - Squamous cell hyperplasia is secondary to chronic irritation (usually recurrent vulvovaginal infections)
  - Lichen planus (a systemic disorder) and lichen simplex chronicus are chronic inflammatory processes
- Cystic lesions of the vulva include epidermal, sebaceous, apocrine gland, and Bartholin's duct cysts
- Vulvodynia refers to a syndrome of chronic vulvar pain, which is associated with vulvar dystrophies and infections but may occur without an identifiable physical cause (essential vulvodynia)

Differential Dx

- Vulvar varicosities (in pregnancy)
- Nevi
- Systemic disorders (e.g., eczema, SLE, psoriasis, scleroderma, pemphigus vulgaris, Behçet syndrome)
- Staphylococcal infections (e.g., impetigo, folliculitis, furunculosis, hidradenitis)
- Pudendal tuberculosis
- Radiation fibrosis
- Malignancy

Presentation

- May be asymptomatic
- Lesions may be noted by patient or upon routine exam
- Vulvar pruritis is the most common symptomatic presentation
  - Itching may be intense and may lead to ulcerations secondary to scratching
- Vulvar pain
- Dyspareunia

Diagnosis/Evaluation

- Biopsy is the standard of diagnosis to rule out malignancy; colposcopy is useful to select the best site for biopsy (5% of patients with a vulvar dystrophy have an underlying malignancy)
- Genital ulcers suggest an infectious etiology and should prompt a workup for sexually transmitted infections
- Essential vulvodynia is a clinical diagnosis made after other causes of vulvar pain have been excluded

Treatment

- Contact dermatitis is treated by removal of the offending agent, cotton underwear, and avoiding tight garments
- Infections should be treated with appropriate antibiotics
- Symptomatic treatment of vulvar dystrophies
  - Lichen sclerosus requires a high-potency steroid; testosterone and/or progestin creams are not effective
  - Squamous cell hyperplasia, lichen simplex chronicus, and lichen planus require medium-potency steroid creams; antihistamines may be added for pruritis
- Cysts generally do not require treatment; incision and drainage may be indicated for large, bothersome, or infected cysts; Bartholin's cysts should be marsupialized to prevent recurrences
- Treatment of vulvodynia should be directed at the cause
  - Symptomatic relief by Sitz baths, topical anesthetics and lubricants, amitriptyline, biofeedback, pain management
  - Refractory cases may require surgery (vestibuloplasty, partial or total vestibulectomy)

Prognosis/Complications

- Vulvar dystrophies are chronic conditions; however, local therapy is successful in 75% of cases
  - Refractory cases may be complicated by introital obstruction and adhesion formation that necessitates surgical intervention
  - 4–6% of patients will develop associated neoplasia
- Secondary infections complicate cysts; occasionally, recurrent abscesses may occur
- 65–70% of patients with vulvodynia find relief with medical therapies; surgical treatment has a variable success rate and some cases persist even after excision

30. Sexually Transmitted Diseases Overview

Etiology/Pathophysiology

- Sexually transmitted diseases (STDs) may be classified by the type of pathogen (bacterial, viral, protozoal, and parasitic)
- There are more than 25 organisms known to be transmitted via sexual contact
- In the past decade, the incidence of bacterial disease has decreased in industrialized nations, but remain epidemic in many parts of the world
- Viral infections are extremely common in the U.S. and worldwide
- Infections are transmitted more effectively from men to women (the vagina serves as a reservoir for pathogens, trauma in intercourse aids transmission)
- In general, populations at risk include teens and young adults
    - More than half of all Americans will acquire at least one lifetime infection
    - The classic bacterial STDs are more frequent in low socioeconomic populations and those with high rates of partner turnover
    - Viral STDs (e.g., HPV) occur frequently in all sexually active populations
- Indications for testing include a history of multiple sex partners, a partner with multiple contacts, sexual contact with someone with an STD, prior history of an STD, and screening is indicated for chlamydia and gonorrhea in all sexually active adolescents and women at high risk of infection

Differential Dx

- Gonorrhea
- Chlamydia
- Syphilis
- Chancroid
- Herpes (HSV)
- Genital warts (HPV)
- Molluscum contagiosum
- Trichomoniasis

Presentation

- Many cases are asymptomatic
- Genital ulcers occur with chancroid, HSV, and syphilis (classic chancre)
- Cervicitis/urethritis occurs with chlamydia and gonorrhea (GC)
- Vaginal discharge/vaginitis occurs with trichomoniasis
- Warts occur with HPV and molluscum contagiosum

Diagnosis/Evaluation

- Thorough sexual history
- Physical exam includes examination of internal and external genitalia, skin, lymph nodes, oropharynx, and perineum
- Site-specific specimens may be collected for specific testing
    - For gonorrhea and chlamydia, swabs are taken from the endocervix or urethra (in women without a cervix); the organisms are detected by Gram stain, culture, or DNA assays
    - Vaginal wet preps are diagnostic of trichomonads
    - Dark field microscopy of pus from a lesion will demonstrate treponemes in primary syphilis
    - Serologic testing for HIV, syphilis, and hepatitis
- Additionally, the anus and oropharynx should be examined if these areas have been exposed to sexual contact
- Screen all pregnant women for STDs and treat appropriately to prevent neonatal infection
- Patients with STD should be offered screening and counseling for HIV (see *Human Immunodeficiency Virus* entry)

Treatment

- Single dose treatments for many STDs are effective and ensure compliance and confidentiality
- Sexual partners should be offered testing and treatment; state health agencies will assist in confidential partner notification; reporting of many STDs is required by law
- Examine all STD patients for concurrent infections
- Gonorrhea and chlamydia must be treated concurrently
- Non-complicated gonorrhea is treated with cefixime (PO), ceftriaxone (IM), or a flouroquinolone (PO); cephalosporins are the treatment of choice in pregnancy
- Chlamydia may be treated with single dose azithromycin or a 7-day course of doxycyline; in pregnancy, amoxicillin or erythromycin is recommended
- Primary and secondary syphilis is treated by a single IM dose of penicillin G; serologic follow up at 6 and 12 months to document cure (doxycylcine if penicillin allergy; if pregnant, desensitize and treat with penicillin)

Prognosis/Complications

- Sequelae (except for HIV) may be avoided if detected early and treated appropriately
- Untreated gonorrhea may disseminate to a dermatitis-arthritis syndrome (0.5–3%)
- Untreated, chlamydia and gonorrhea can infect the upper genital tract, causing PID and/or inflammation of liver capsule (peri-hepatitis or Fitz-Hugh-Curtis syndrome)
- Chlamydia conjunctivitis may occur via auto-inoculation; neonatal infection (conjunctivitis and pneumonia) may occur via an infected birth canal
- Untreated syphilis may result in secondary syphilis (rash, lymphadenopathy), tertiary syphilis (gummas, neurosyphilis, aortic aneurysms, valvular insufficiencies), and congenital syphilis (may be fatal)

31. Pelvic Inflammatory Disease

Etiology/Pathophysiology

- Pelvic inflammatory disease (PID) results from ascending infection and subsequent inflammation of the upper female genital tract
- The most common organisms that cause pelvic inflammatory disease are *Neisseria gonorrhoeae* and *Chlamydia trachomatis* (2/3 have one or both); *Mycoplasma hominis*, *Ureaplasma urealyticum*, Group B strep, anaerobes, and gram negatives are also implicated in some cases
- Most commonly, PID occurs secondary to sexually transmitted infections; however, it may also occur following instrumentation of the uterus
- Approximately 10% of women will develop PID during their reproductive years and a significant number of these patients will have complications; PID often goes undiagnosed because some cases are asymptomatic or have mild nonspecific signs or symptoms

Differential Dx

- Appendicitis
- Ectopic pregnancy
- Ovarian cyst (rupture or torsion)
- Mittelschmerz (ovulatory pain)
- Endometriosis
- Renal/urethral stone
- UTI/pyelonephritis
- Bowel pathology

Presentation

- Low abdominal pain
- Cervical motion tenderness
- Adnexal and uterine tenderness
- Dyspareunia (especially if recent onset)
- Mucopurulent cervical discharge
- Fever, nausea, vomiting
- Elevated WBCs, sedimentation rate, and C-reactive protein
- May be asymptomatic (especially if caused by *Chlamydia*)

Diagnosis/Evaluation

- CDC diagnostic criteria suggest the need to initiate empiric treatment (in order to reduce a missed diagnosis of PID, which may result in damage to the reproductive tract): In women who are sexually active and at risk of infection, initiate treatment if all three minimal criteria are met (additional criteria support the diagnosis of PID); however, it is not necessary to establish definitive criteria before treating
- Minimal criteria: Lower abdominal tenderness, cervical motion tenderness, or adnexal tenderness
- Additional criteria include oral temperature >38.3° C (101° F), abnormal cervical or vaginal discharge; elevated ESR; elevated C-reactive protein, and lab documentation of cervical gonorrhea or chlamydia infection
- Definitive criteria
    - Endometritis on endometrial biopsy
    - Transvaginal ultrasound reveals thickened fluid-filled tubes with or without free pelvic fluid or tubo-ovarian complex
    - Findings on laparoscopy consistent with PID

Treatment

- Antibiotic coverage should cover all possible organisms
- Outpatient treatment is available for non-complicated cases:
    - Ofloxacin plus metronidazole for 14 days
    - Third-generation cepahalosporin (single dose) plus doxycycline for 14 days
- If there is no response to oral antibiotics within 72 hours, the patient should be admitted for re-evaluation and parenteral antibiotics
    - Parenteral regimens include cefotetan or cefoxitin plus doxycycline; clindamycin plus gentamicin; or a fluoroquinolone plus metronidazole
    - Patients may be switched to oral therapy if afebrile for 24 hours
- Other indications for hospitalization include patients who are severely ill on presentation, pregnant patients, and patients with tubo-ovarian abscess

Prognosis/Complications

- The major complications of PID are tubal damage and adhesion formation
- Infertility may occur secondary to damage of the tubal epithelium; the incidence of infertility increases with each episode of PID
    - 1 episode: 8% risk
    - 2 episodes: 20% risk
    - 3+ episodes: 40% risk
- The incidence of ectopic pregnancy increases 10-fold after PID
- Adhesions may lead to chronic pelvic pain and dyspareunia

32. Human Papilloma Virus

Etiology/Pathophysiology

- Human papilloma viruses (HPV) infect epithelial tissues and are spread via sexual contact
- HPV infection is extremely common
  - In sexually active populations, the prevalence may be 50% or more
  - Most sexually active women will be exposed at least once during their lives
- HPV is most often asymptomatic and self-limited (6–12 months) but may present with genital warts (condyloma acuminatum)
  - Asymptomatic transmission is common
- There are over 25 HPV serotypes that have been isolated from the female genital tract; some serotypes have been causally associated with precancerous and cancerous lesions of the cervix (16 and 18 are most common; other high-risk types include 31, 33, 35, and 45)
- Risk factors include early age of sexual activity, multiple sex partners, sex with an uncircumcised partner, and co-infection with other STDs
- Risk factors for cervical disease include all the risk factors for infection plus longer duration of infection, and high viral load
- Immunosuppression is associated with higher rates of infection and severity of disease

Differential Dx

- Condyloma lata (secondary syphilis)
- Molluscum contagiosum
- Seborrheic keratosis
- Lichen planus
- Neoplastic lesions

Presentation

- The majority of infections are asymptomatic
- Patients will present when they notice the appearance of a lesion (genital wart)
- Warts typically occur in and around the introitus and on the labia; they may also exist on the cervix, vagina, clitoris, urethra, and anus
- Cervical lesions may cause spotting and post-coital bleeding

Diagnosis/Evaluation

- Warts are diagnosed by history and the characteristic appearance of the lesion (well-circumscribed, raised warty lesion on an otherwise healthy vulva); if necessary, biopsy will confirm the diagnosis
- For cervical lesions, application of acetic acid followed by colposcopy will demonstrate the characteristic "acetowhitening" of HPV-infected areas
- PCR and hybrid capture assays may be used to isolate HPV and for serotyping
- Pap smears are used to screen women for precancerous changes associated with HPV infection
  - Findings include koilocytosis, atypical squamous cells of uncertain significance (ASCUS), squamous intra-epithelial lesion of low grade (LGSIL) or high grade (HGSIL), and carcinoma in situ
- HPV testing is a triage option in the management of an initial ASCUS Pap
  - Negative findings eliminate the need for more invasive tests
  - Testing is essential for recurrent ASCUS lesions

Treatment

- Asymptomatic disease may not require treatment
- Warts should be removed with attention to cosmetic outcome
  - 0.5% podofilox solution or gel applied to warts by the patient BID for 3 days, followed by 4 days without therapy; this cycle may be repeated up to 4 times
  - 5% imiquimod cream applied to warts by the patient 3 times per week for 16 weeks
  - Provider-applied treatments include cryotherapy (liquid nitrogen or cryoprobe), 10–25% podophyllin resin in tincture of benzoin, 80–90% trichloracetic acid, intra-lesional interferon, and surgical removal (via tangential scissor excision, shave excision, curettage, electrosurgery, or laser surgery)
- See *Evaluation of an Abnormal Pap Smear* entry
- HPV vaccines are currently being developed; early research in animal models has been promising and human trials are under way

Prognosis/Complications

- Data on outcomes of asymptomatic HPV infection are limited; many cases are never diagnosed
- Treatment does not eliminate infection nor alter the natural history of disease
- Symptomatic partners should be treated
- For warts, response depends on the immune status of the patient and the number, size, and location of lesions
- Up to two-thirds of patients will have a recurrence of warts 6–12 weeks after treatment is stopped; however, most will resolve within a year
- If warts are resistant to treatment, consider biopsy to rule out malignancy
- Within 2 years, 68% of ASCUS lesions, 47% of LGSIL lesions, and 35% of HGSIL lesions will return to normal

33. Herpes Simplex Virus

Etiology/Pathophysiology

- Herpes infection of the genital tract is one of the most common viral STDs
- The initial genital infection due to herpes may be asymptomatic or associated with severe symptoms
  - Symptomatic primary infection results in lesions on the vulva, vagina, or cervix 2–14 days following exposure
  - When systemic symptoms (malaise, myalgia, and fever) occur, they are most commonly restricted to presumed primary herpetic infections, reflecting the viremia that often occurs
- Recurrences of genital HSV infections can be symptomatic or subclinical; ulcers tend to be limited in size, number, and duration
- Subclinical shedding can occur without symptoms or signs of clinical lesions, making this viral STD difficult to control and prevent
- Infection is caused by herpes simplex viruses HSV-1 and HSV-2
  - Both viruses are transmitted by sexual contact
  - HSV-2 causes more frequent outbreaks and has a greater degree of asymptomatic shedding
- Like other herpes virus infections, HSV lives and replicates in nerve ganglia and causes recurrent outbreaks in the skin and mucosa

Differential Dx

- Other diseases that cause genital ulcers
  - Chancroid
  - HSV
  - Primary syphilis (classic chancre)
  - Lymphogranuloma venereum (LGV)
  - Granuloma inguinale
  - Behçet's disease
  - Genital trauma
  - Vulvar cancer

Presentation

- Primary HSV lasts 3 weeks and is severe
  - Papules form vesicles, which break to form ulcers, and then crust over and heal; often painful and/or itchy
  - Dysuria and urinary retention may be present
  - May also present as cervicitis
  - Mild systemic symptoms (e.g., fever, malaise) may be present
- Recurrent infection is milder, with fewer lesions or small linear ulcerations, and lasts <1 week
- In some cases, the initial presentation may resemble a recurrent infection

Diagnosis/Evaluation

- Generally a clinical diagnosis
- Viral culture, antigen detection, serology, and/or PCR may be used and all have high sensitivity
- Tzanck prep may be used to identify the characteristic multi-nucleated giant cells; this test is easy and cheap, but is only 50% sensitive
- Blood tests for seropositivity are not useful; studies do indicate that some patients who are seropositive are never symptomatic, but are still shedding virus and are infectious

Treatment

- Goals of therapy are to decrease the duration and frequency of outbreaks and to lessen the risk of transmission to partners
- Treatment is with thymidine kinase-dependent antivirals, including acyclovir, valacyclovir, and famciclovir
  - Episodic treatment will abort outbreaks in 25% of cases, if started during the prodrome; if the outbreak is not aborted, healing time occurs more rapidly and shedding is decreased
  - Daily suppressive therapy may be used in an attempt to reduce the frequency of outbreaks; daily therapy is indicated in patients with more than six outbreaks/year
- Antiviral therapy for primary infection is recommended for pregnant women with primary HSV infection to reduce viral shedding and enhance lesion healing, for suppressive therapy for the duration of pregnancy to reduce the potential of viral shedding, and for management of women with recurrent HSV in pregnancy

Prognosis/Complications

- Recurrences usually occur 2–6 times/year; 90% infected with HSV-2 will have at least one outbreak in the first year, 35% of patients will have six or more outbreaks
- HSV-1 causes fewer outbreaks
- 50% of reactivations are asymptomatic, but patients still have viral shedding and can transmit the virus
- Patients with co-existent HIV infection have more severe disease and increased viral shedding; ulcers may be chronic and superinfected with bacteria
- 30–50% risk of neonatal transmission through an infected birth canal in primary HSV disease, 3% risk during recurrent episodes; C-section reduces the risk and is recommended at onset of labor if signs and symptoms of infection are present

34. Human Immunodeficiency Virus

Etiology/Pathophysiology

- Human immunodeficiency virus (HIV) is a member of the lentivirus family of retroviruses
- Primarily contracted through intimate sexual contact (genital-genital, genital-anal, genital-oral); perinatal transmission from mother to child; and use of contaminated needles or blood products
- HIV infection can be transmitted perinatally across the placenta, during delivery, or through breast milk; the risk of transmission is proportional to the maternal viral load
- The main risk factor for HIV transmission to women is heterosexual contact
- Primary HIV infection: To enter the cell, the HIV envelope protein GP-120 binds to the CD4 molecule of dendritic cells; HIV-infected cells fuse with CD4+ lymphocytes and the virus spreads; acute retroviral syndrome develops (resulting in flu-like symptoms); partial immunity develops and can be maintained for several years
- Acquired immune deficiency syndrome (AIDS) is caused by HIV
  - Occurs when the CD4 count is below 200/mL
  - Characterized by the appearance of opportunistic infections

Differential Dx

- Primary infection
  - Mononucleosis (Epstein-Barr virus)
  - Cytomegalovirus
  - Toxoplasmosis
  - Rubella
  - Syphilis
  - Viral hepatitis
  - New onset systemic lupus erythematosis
- AIDS
  - Malnutrition
  - Hereditary immunodeficiencies
  - Acquired immunodeficiencies

Presentation

- HIV testing should be recommended to all sexually active persons and those with high-risk behaviors during routine health maintenance exams
- Patients with asymptomatic primary HIV infection often do not seek medical attention
- Symptoms of primary HIV infection include fever, sore throat, diarrhea, weight loss, lymphadenopathy, mucocutaneous lesions, and myalgias/arthralgias
- Patients may present with opportunistic infections or illnesses reflecting their immunodeficient state:
  - *Mycobacterium avium* infection
  - *Pneumocystis carinii* pneumonia
  - Kaposi's sarcoma

Diagnosis/Evaluation

- Perform a thorough history and examination (especially for rash, mucocutaneous ulcers, and lymphadenopathy)
- Enzyme-linked immunosorbent assay (ELISA) detects serum antibodies to HIV; however, ELISA does result in false positives, so confirm positive ELISA tests with a Western blot
- Test viral load and CD4 count at diagnosis, every 3–4 months for patients not on therapy, 2–8 weeks after beginning therapy, and every 3–4 months while on therapy
- Genotype testing at diagnosis to establish drug resistance
- Test for IgG antibody to *Toxoplasma* to detect latent infection
- Check tuberculosis skin test
- Counsel on need for barrier protection with sexual activity (reduces transmission by 85%); protection needed even with HAART therapy (see below) and undetectable viral load
- Universal screening for HIV in pregnancy with patient notification is a routine component of prenatal care; early diagnosis allows effective retrovirus therapy for maternal health and reduced risk of neonatal transmission

Treatment

- Offer treatment to all patients with HIV symptoms and to those with CD4 counts ≤350/μL or HIV RNA levels ≥55,000 copies/mL
- HAART: two nucleoside reverse transcriptase inhibitors (e.g., zidovudine, didanosine, lamivudine) plus one protease inhibitor (e.g., indinavir, ritinavir) or one non-nucleoside reverse transcriptase inhibitor (e.g., nevirapine)
- After 16–20 weeks of therapy, the viral load should be undetectable (≤50 RNA copies/mL) and remain low
- If viral loads do not decrease or rise, change the regimen
- Zidovudine prophylaxis during pregnancy, labor, and for the newborn reduces the risk of perinatal transmission by 70% (continue HAART if already on the regimen)
- Women with viral loads ≥100,000 RNA copies/mL should be counseled regarding cesarean delivery before the onset of labor or rupture of membranes to reduce transmission beyond that of retroviral therapy alone

Prognosis/Complications

- Development of opportunistic infections includes *P. carinii* pneumonia (CD4 count ≤ 200/μL), *Toxoplasma* encephalitis (CD4 count ≤ 100/μL), *M. avium* complex (CD4 count ≤ 50/μL), candida esophagitis, and vaginitis
- Abnormal Pap tests and neurologic complications may occur
- Risks of therapy include symptomatic and long-term toxicities, drug resistance, nausea, vomiting, fatigue, and hepatotoxicity
- Pregnancy does not appear to accelerate HIV progression or maternal mortality
- Breastfeeding is contraindicated in maternal HIV infection because of the risk of transmission

35. Toxic Shock Syndrome

Etiology/Pathophysiology

- Syndrome of multi-organ system failure, hypotension, fever, and rash
- TSS is caused by colonization or infection with specific strains of *Staphylococcus aureus* that produce the epidermal toxin toxic shock syndrome toxin-1 (TSST-1) and other enterotoxins
- First described in a series of pediatric cases in 1978
- The incidence rose in 1980 in young white women, associated with the use of highly absorbent tampons
- Withdrawal of highly absorbent tampons and polyacrylate rayon-containing products from the market has led to decrease in menses-related TSS, from 9 to 1 out of 100,000 women since 1986
- Currently, 59% of TSS is of menstrual origin (41% of nonmenstrual origin)
- Variant of TSS described in patients with AIDS
- Risk factors
  - Menstrual TSS: Use of tampons with higher absorbencies, continuously for more days, or a single tampon in place for a longer period of time
  - Nonmenstrual TSS: Surgery and postpartum wound infections, mastitis, septorhinoplasty, sinusitis, osteomyelitis, arthritis, burns, cutaneous and subcutaneous lesions, influenza respiratory infections

Differential Dx

- Streptococcal toxic shock syndrome
- Rocky Mountain spotted fever
- Meningococcemia
- Meningitis
- Leptospirosis
- Dengue hemorrhagic fever
- Typhoid fever
- Sepsis
- Viral syndrome

Presentation

- Symptoms develop rapidly in otherwise healthy women
- Median interval between menstruation onset/post-surgical and TSS: 2–3 days
- Onset of symptoms may be as late as 65 days postoperatively
- Fever >38.8°C (102°F)
- Hypotension
- Rash: Diffuse macular erythroderma
- Desquamation 1–2 weeks after onset of illness, particularly palms and soles
- Myalgias, weakness
- Disorientation, confusion, seizure; headaches, memory loss, poor concentration
- Other: Pulmonary edema, pleural effusions, depression of myocardial function, hepatic dysfunction, anemia, thrombocytopenia

Diagnosis/Evaluation

- Multisystem involvement (3+ organ systems)
  - GI: Vomiting, diarrhea at illness onset
  - Muscular: Severe myalgia or elevated CPK
  - Renal: BUN/creatinine elevation or pyuria
  - Hepatic: Elevated bilirubin or transaminases
  - Hematologic: Platelets <100,000/μL
  - CNS: Disoriented, altered consciousness without focal neurologic signs
- Cultures from mucosal and wound sites may be used for confirmation but are not necessary for diagnosis
- *S. aureus* is rarely recovered from blood cultures, possibly because the exotoxin is absorbed through the vaginal mucosa

Treatment

- Hospitalization is required due to the seriousness of the disease, intensive care unit may be necessary for hemodynamic instability
- Supportive therapy: Extensive fluid replacement, pressor agents
- Surgical therapy: Removal of infectious foreign material if present
- Antibiotic therapy: Clindamycin, plus oxacillin or nafcillin (does not shorten course of illness, but may prevent recurrence)
- Additional therapies: IV immunoglobulin, corticosteroids
- Preventive measures include limiting highly absorbent tampon use to days of heavy flow, or interchange with pads

Prognosis/Complications

- Menses-related TSS may resolve with supportive therapy only
- Prerenal and intrinsic renal failure can occur accompanied by hyponatremia, hypoalbuminemia, hypocalcemia, and hypophosphatemia
- Recurrence may occur in patients not treated with appropriate courses of antibiotics or if patient fails to develop an appropriate antibody response
- Recurrence may occur days to months after the initial episode
- 30% risk of menstrual TSS in women who resume use of high-absorbency tampons

36. Female Sexual Dysfunction

Etiology/Pathophysiology

- WHO definition of FSD: The various ways in which an individual is unable to participate in a sexual relationship as he or she would wish
- DSM IV definition of FSD: Disturbances in sexual desire and in the psychophysiologic changes that characterize the sexual response cycle and cause marked distress and interpersonal difficulties
- 1998 Consensus Panel: The diagnosis of FSD requires that the dysfunction cause "personal distress" and each of the sexual dysfunction diagnoses is independent of all of the others
- Recent studies report a prevalence of 20–50%; American Urological Association frequently cites 43%
- >90% of women seeking routine gynecologic care report ≥1 sexual concern
- Most frequent types of sexual dysfunction: Hypoactive sexual desire, sexual arousal disorder, orgasmic disorder, lubrication difficulties, and dyspareunia
- Risk factors: Genital atrophy; sexual abuse; psychological factors; interpersonal or relationship disorders; peripheral vascular, cardiovascular, or neurologic disease; endocrinopathies; life stressors; medications (e.g., antidepressants, OCPs, anti-androgens, anti-estrogens, anticholinergics, antihistamines); hysterectomy; breast or gynecologic malignancies

Differential Dx

- Hypoactive sexual desire disorder
- Sexual aversion disorder
- Sexual arousal disorder
- Orgasmic disorder
- Sexual pain disorders
    −Dyspareunia
    −Vaginismus
- Non-coital sexual pain disorder
- Psychological causes
- Medication side effects
- Failure of genital response
- Systemic medical or surgical condition that affects sexual function

Presentation

- Only 10–20% of afflicted women seek medical consultation
- Fewer women volunteer a history of FSD during routine medical visits
- Based on personal history complaints range, from decreased desire, poor lubrication, sensation and/or orgasmic potential, to pain with stimulation or upon penetration
- Women often report a change from their previous baseline sexual function and satisfaction or a concern or difficulty in an area of their sexual life, not previously experienced

Diagnosis/Evaluation

- Diagnosis begins with physician actively eliciting the information as part of the routine medical history, including questions regarding sexual interest, arousal, orgasm, and pain
- Physical examination, including a pelvic examination, seeking evidence of vaginal atrophy, dryness, causes of pain or dyspareunia, and pain-triggering areas
- Consultation with a sexual therapist for psychosocial evaluation and sexual education
- The recently validated female sexual function index (FSFI) self-report questionnaire is used to monitor treatment efficacy, and it assesses specific domains including desire, lubrication, and orgasm
- Endocrinological evaluation includes serum FSH, LH, estradiol, DHEAS, total and free testosterone, and prolactin
- Clinical evaluation of FSD includes measuring vaginal pH, genital blood flow via Doppler ultrasound, vaginal wall compliance, clitoral and vaginal temperature and oxygenation, and genital vibratory perception/sensation thresholds (available in specialized centers)

Treatment

- Treat underlying physiologic disorders, if present
- Patient education and maximization of physical health
- Avoid medications known to cause FSD
- FDA-approved EROS clitoral therapy device: Vacuum device increases cavernosal blood flow, engorgement, and vaginal lubrication; effective in women with arousal and orgasmic difficulties
- Sildenafil has been variably effective; reverses side effects of loss of sexual interest, anorgasmic of SSRI use, and women with spinal cord injuries
- Hormone replacement improves urogenital atrophy and vasomotor symptoms
- Administer exogenous androgen for women with known androgen and arousal disorders
- Testosterone replacement therapy may be used for disorders of desire; no consensus on therapeutic levels; may have a role in testosterone deficient or oophorectomized women

Prognosis/Complications

- Research on FSD is proceeding rapidly and the underlying physiologic processes in "normal" and "dysfunctional" sexual function are being defined
- New treatment options require further evaluation with randomized clinical trials using larger sample sizes and longer duration of follow up
- A multidisciplinary approach to the treatment of FSD, including the physical, psychosocial, and relationship aspects, appears most promising at present
- Current treatment options such as testosterone replacement in women, are not without risk (may cause hepatic disease, polycythemia, alopecia, acne, hirsutism) and the risk-benefit ratio must be analyzed individually; no data in breast cancer

37. Infertility

Etiology/Pathophysiology

- Definition: Failure to conceive after 1 year of regular unprotected intercourse; most clinicians start a workup at 6 months for women 35 or older
- Fecundity naturally 20% each cycle, 50% at 3 months, 85% at 1 year
- 1 in 6 couples have infertility and it is more common with increasing age
- Male factors (40% of cases)
  - Endocrine disorders: Pituitary/hypothalamic dysfunction, adrenal hyperplasia, thyroid disease, testosterone deficiency
  - Abnormal spermatogenesis: Mumps orchitis, varicocele, cryptorchidism
  - Abnormal motility: Antisperm antibodies, immotile cilia syndrome
  - Sexual dysfunction: Retrograde ejaculation, impotence, ductal obstruction
- Female factors (40% of cases)
  - Peritoneal factors (40%): Pelvic adhesions from prior surgery, endometriosis, and chronic PID
  - Ovulatory factors (15–20%): Polycystic ovarian syndrome, thyroid dysfunction, premature ovarian failure
  - Uterine-tubal factors (30%): Tubal occlusion, fibroids, endometriosis
  - Cervical factors (5–10%): Structural abnormalities, mucus abnormalities
- Unexplained (20% of cases)

Differential Dx

- Pituitary/hypothalamic dysfunction
- Thyroid disease
- Endometriosis
- Tubal occlusion
- Chronic PID
- Pelvic adhesions
- Fibroids
- Antisperm antibodies
- Retrograde ejaculation
- Impotence
- Varicocele
- Cryptorchidism
- Immotile cilia
- Mumps orchitis
- Asherman syndrome
- Carcinoma

Presentation

- Male factor infertility: May present with lack of sexual hair growth; gynecomastia; varicocele; scars of hernia repair or trauma to genitals; hypogonadism
- Female factor infertility: May present with dysmenorrhea or cyclic pelvic pain, dyspareunia, and menstrual irregularity outside the normal range (22–35 days); hirsutism, obesity, galactorrhea, or signs of virilism; recurrent pregnancy loss, heavy bleeding, and pain; signs of thyroid disease; may have history of prior cryotherapy, conization, or cervical dilations

Diagnosis/Evaluation

- Complete medical history and physical examination looking for risk factors that could affect fertility
- Tests for male factor: Semen analysis: Sperm count, volume, motility, morphology, pH, WBC count; if results abnormal (especially if <10 mil/mL sperm), follow up with endocrine tests (FSH, testosterone, TSH, prolactin); less common tests include postejaculatory urinalysis (if semen volume <1.0 mL) to look for retrograde ejaculation, and post-coital test of interaction between sperm and cervical mucus
- Tests for female factor: Ovulatory-endocrine evaluation includes menstrual history, basal body temperature charts, FSH on day 21 (>3 ng/mL is confirmatory), urine LH surge (ovulatory predictor kits), TSH, and prolactin; in women 35 or older, test for FSH on day 3 (assesses ovarian reserve); uterine-tubal evaluation includes a hystersalpingogram to see if the uterine cavity and fallopian tubes are normal in size and shape; peritoneal examination via laparoscopy if there is a history of increasing dysmenorrhea

Treatment

- Male factor
  - Correction of endocrine disorders
  - Limit intercourse to once every 2 days
  - Repair of anatomic defects (varicocele)
  - Washed sperm for intrauterine insemination
  - Intracytoplasmic sperm injection (ICSI)
  - Refractory cases: Artificial insemination with donor sperm
- Female factor
  - Intrauterine insemination (IUI)
  - Ovulation induction with clomiphene citrate or gonadotropins
  - In vitro fertilization (IVF) or gamete intrafallopian transfer (GIFT) and gonadotropins
  - Refractory cases: Egg or embryo donation, gestational surrogacy, or adoption

Prognosis/Complications

- Correction of endocrine disorders generally restores fertility
- Surgical ligation of varicoceles restores fertility in 50% of cases
- Clomiphene is associated with multiple pregnancy (8–10%), ovarian cysts (5–10%)
- Gonadotropin therapy is associated with multiple pregnancy (33%), and ovarian hyperstimulation syndrome (1.3%)
- IVF is associated with multiple pregnancy (38%), ovarian hyperstimulation (5%), and increased pregnancy losses (25%) and ectopic pregnancy (5%)
- Pregnancy rate in unexplained, untreated infertility cases approaches 60% over 3–5 years

38. Spontaneous & Recurrent Abortions

Etiology/Pathophysiology

- Spontaneous abortion (SAB): A pregnancy that ends before 20 weeks gestation; it is estimated that 15–25% of all pregnancies end in SAB
- Recurrent abortion: Two, three, or more consecutive pregnancy losses
  - <1% of the population is affected
  - Risk of recurrence after one prior SAB is 20–25%; after two consecutive SABs is 25–30%; and after three consecutive SABs is 30–35%
  - A live birth reduces the risk of SAB in the subsequent gestation
- Etiology
  - Genetic (60–80% of first trimester SABs): Autosomal trisomy, monosomy X
  - Anatomic: Uterine malformations, intrauterine adhesions, fibroids, incompetent cervix
  - Endocrine (15–60% of RSABs): Polycystic ovary syndrome, thyroid disease, poorly controlled diabetes, hyperprolactinemia, luteal phase defect
  - Immunologic: Anti-phospholipid antibody (APA) syndrome (results in 15% of all cases of recurrent SAB), SLE
  - Environmental: Smoking, alcohol, chemicals, radiation
  - Infectious: Bacteria, mycoplasma, viruses
  - Over 1/3 of all cases of recurrent SABs are unexplained

Differential Dx

- Threatened abortion
- Ectopic pregnancy
- Molar pregnancy
- Incompetent cervix
- Vaginal/cervical lesion
- Fibroids

Presentation

- Vaginal bleeding
- Cramping and abdominal pain
- Decreased symptoms of pregnancy
- Threatened abortion: Painless vaginal bleeding with closed cervix
- Inevitable abortion: Cervix is dilated, bleeding is increasing with strong uterine contractions/cramps
- Incomplete abortion: Cervix is open with partial expulsion of some, but not all products of conception (POC); bleeding may be severe
- Missed abortion: Inutero death of the embryo or fetus with retained POC
- Septic abortion: Fever, chills, malaise, abdominal pain, vaginal bleeding, and often a purulent discharge

Diagnosis/Evaluation

- Complete history and physical exam
- Pelvic exam: Look for sources of bleeding other than uterine
  - Vaginal bleeding is common in the first trimester (22%) and is not always associated with impending abortion
- Cervical changes: Closed, softened, dilated, presence of POC
- Labs should include a quantitative β-hCG, CBC, blood typing, and antibody screen
- Ultrasound is used to assess fetal viability and placentation
- Rule out ectopic pregnancy
- Begin recurrent SAB evaluation after the second SAB
  - Karyotype of both parents and POC
  - Uterine assessment using sonohysterography, or hysterosalpingography
  - Anticardiolipin antibodies, lupus anticoagulant
  - Endometrial biopsy is controversial (assess for luteal phase defect)

Treatment

- Hypotensive or hemorrhaging patients must be stabilized; administer RhoGAM to all Rh-negative patients with bleeding
- Threatened abortions: Follow for continued bleeding and place on pelvic rest with nothing per vagina
- Inevitable, incomplete, and missed abortions: Dilation and evacuation, expectant management, or misoprostol to expedite the expulsion of the products of contraception; follow bleeding; high-dose oxytocin or prostaglandins will induce labor (16–24 weeks gestation)
- Abnormal karyotype: IVF with pre-implantation genetic diagnosis, gamete donation, surrogacy, or adoption
- Uterine pathology: Surgery for correctable causes
- Irreparable uterine defects: Surrogacy or adoption
- Cervical incompetence: Cervical cerclage placement
- APA syndrome: Low-dose aspirin with low-dose heparin
- Polycystic ovary syndrome: Metformin

Prognosis/Complications

- Prognosis for having a successful future pregnancy after an SAB or recurrent SAB is good
- Recurrent SABs remain unexplained in over 1/3 of couples
- The chance of having a live birth after three unexplained recurrent SABs is still 50–70% even without intervention

39. Assisted Reproduction

Indications

- Ovulatory dysfunction
  - With normal FSH and prolactin levels: Ovulation induction with clomiphene citrate (anti-estrogen)
  - With hypothalamic/pituitary dysfunction or failed clomiphene citrate: Ovulation induction with human menopausal gonadotropin (FSH/LH) or recombinant FSH
- Endometriosis: Ovulation induction preceded by suppression with danocrine, or leuprolide acetate; in vitro fertilization (IVF), zygote intrafallopian transfer (ZIFT), or gamete intrafallopian transfer (GIFT) in mild cases
- Cervical factor infertility: Intrauterine insemination (IUI)
- Tubal factor infertility: IVF
- Antisperm antibodies: IUI, IVF, GIFT, or ZIFT
- Male factor infertility: IUI if defect is mild (e.g., oligospermia, high semen viscosity, etc); for severe cases, intracytoplasmic sperm injection (ICSI) and IVF, or GIFT combined with ICSI, or ZIFT
- Unexplained infertility: IUI, IVF, GIFT or ZIFT

Epidemiology

- Types of assisted reproduction used in the U.S.
  - 97% IVF
  - 1% GIFT
  - 1% ZIFT
- Assisted reproduction diagnosis in the U.S.
  - 40% male factor
  - 16% tubal factor
  - 7% endometriosis
  - 5% ovulatory dysfunction
  - 1% uterine factor
  - 7% other
  - 20% unexplained

Side Effects

- Clomiphene citrate: Nausea, insomnia, hot flashes, depression, emotional lability, headache, and visual changes
- Gonadotropins: Abdominal discomfort, bloating, headache and/or fatigue, and injection site discomfort
- Microsurgical epididymal sperm aspiration: Infection
- IUI: Cramping and bleeding
- IVF: Cramping and bleeding
- GIFT: Abdominal and/or laparoscopic incision site discomfort, cramping, and bleeding
- ZIFT: Abdominal and/or laparoscopic incision site discomfort, cramping. and bleeding

Alternative Treatments

- Adoption
- Gestational surrogacy
- Ovulation induction (clomiphene citrate or gonadotropins)
- Expectant management (using higher technological alternatives, which are uncommonly used)
- Pre-implantation genetic diagnosis (PGD) for known carriers of specific genetic defects
- ICSI for low sperm density or impaired motility, followed by IVF or GIFT
- Microsurgical epididymal sperm aspiration (MESA) followed by IVF
- Testicular sperm extraction (TESA) followed by IVF
- IUI
- IVF
- GIFT
- ZIFT
- Donor egg and/or sperm, or donor embryo

Efficacy

- Clomid induces ovulation in 70% of correctly selected patients; 5–38% fecundity per cycle
- IUI in healthy young women has a 15–25% pregnancy rate per cycle
- Gonadotropin has an 85–90% success rate of ovulation induction after six cycles
- GIFT and ZIFT have pregnancy rates of 22–28% per cycle
- IVF with intracytoplasmic sperm injection has pregnancy rates of 20–40% per cycle
- Success rates for IVF in the U.S. (live births per cycle):
  - Fresh non-donor eggs: Women age <35 (32%), 35–37 (26.2%), 38–40 (18.5%), >40 (9.7%)
  - Frozen non-donor eggs: Women age <35 (19.7%), 35–37 (19.1%), 38–40 (15.8%), >40 (16.2%)
  - Fresh donor eggs: Women age <35, 35–37, 38–40, >40 (all similar success rates of 41.6%)

Complications

- Multiple fetal pregnancy, which also increases risk for miscarriage, preterm delivery, and bleeding
  - Clomiphene (8%)
  - Gonadotropin (20%)
  - IVF (38%)
- Ovarian hyperstimulation syndrome is usually mild, but can be severe and life threatening
  - Gonadotropin (1–3%)
- Ectopic pregnancy
  - IVF (4%)
- Flare up of unsuspected pelvic infection
  - Intrauterine insemination
- Birth defects (due to damaged meiotic spindle)
  - Intracytoplasmic sperm injection

40. Abortion

Indications

- Fetal abnormalities
- Pregnancy that puts the mother's life at risk
- Elective pregnancy termination before fetal viability (approximately 24 weeks gestation)
  - Undesired pregnancy
  - Congenital abnormalities
  - Severe hyperemesis
  - Previable preterm premature rupture of membranes
  - Life-threatening maternal condition
- Elective pregnancy termination after 24 weeks gestation
  - Life-threatening maternal condition

Epidemiology

- Approximately 25% of all pregnancies world-wide end in elective abortion
- 1 million abortions are performed annually in the US: 1/3 on women under age 20; 1/3 on women ages 20–24; 1/3 on women >25; about 75% are unmarried women
- Suction curettage is the most common method in the U.S.
- Medical abortion accounts for <1% of all cases

Side Effects

- Mifepristone (RU-486) with misoprostol: Substantial uterine cramping/pain, nausea, vomiting, diarrhea, headache, dizziness, back pain, and tiredness (side effects lessen after day 3 and are usually gone by day 14)
  - Vaginal administration results in fewer side effects than oral
- Induction of labor: Abdominal cramping, vaginal bleeding, nausea, vomiting, diarrhea, and fever
- Menstrual extraction: Abdominal cramping and vaginal bleeding
- Suction curettage: Abdominal cramping
- Dilation and evacuation: Abdominal cramping

Alternative Treatments

- Post-coital pill (within 72 hours of intercourse)
- Continuation of pregnancy
- Adoption
- Medical abortion (limited to pregnancies <50 days of gestation)
  - Methotrexate (blocks dihydrofolate reductase) followed by vaginal misoprostol (prostaglandin E_1 analog)
  - Mifepristone (RU-486) administered orally or vaginally, followed by misoprostol
- Induction of labor: Intrauterine instillation (prostaglandin F_{2a} and hypertonic saline combined) and vaginal prostaglandin E_2 suppositories or oxytocin
- Medical abortion failures should be managed by surgical dilation and evacuation
- Surgical abortion
  - Menstrual extraction (if <7 week gestation)
  - Suction curettage (if <14 weeks gestation)
  - Dilation and evacuation (if beyond 14 weeks of gestation)

Efficacy

- Mifepristone (RU-486) followed after 48 hours with misoprostol: efficacy rate 96% up to 49 days
- Methotrexate and misoprostol has an efficacy rate of 92–96% up to 49 days
- Efficacy rates for both of the above medical abortions declines significantly for gestations over 7 weeks
- Induction of labor: Varies from 80–100% success rate, depending on the regimen used
  - Intrauterine instillation
- Menstrual extraction: Rate of failure is low (0.13%–4%)
- Suction curettage: When performed by a trained physician, the efficacy rate is 98–99%
  - Failures occur at early gestational ages (<7 weeks)
- Dilation and evacuation: High efficacy rate; safer than induction of labor when second trimester termination is necessary

Complications

- Suction curettage (complications are rare): Endometritis, hemorrhage, uterine perforation, hematometra (postabortal syndrome), and anesthesia problems
- Mifepristone and methotrexate: Incomplete or failed abortion, and prolonged heavy uterine bleeding; misoprostol is teratogenic
- Induction of labor (complication rate is high): Retained placenta, incomplete abortion, hemorrhage, coagulopathy, infection, and emotional stress
  - Intravaginal prostaglandins have a high incidence of live births
  - Instillation agents have a high rate of retained placenta
- Dilation and evacuation (complications are uncommon): Hemorrhage, infection, perforation, and retained tissues

41. Sterilization (Male & Female)

Indications

- Surgical procedure to block or remove male or female genital tracts to prevent fertilization
- Female sterilization is via tubal occlusion: Surgically sever and/or occlude the paired fallopian tubes using bands, clips, or by cauterization; not as simple as male sterilization, as tubes are located deep in the pelvis
    - Mini-laparotomy: Commonly performed on postpartum women (preferably within the first 24 hours), morbidly obese, and women with severe tubal adhesive disease
    - Laparoscopy: Commonly performed for interval sterilization (unrelated to pregnancy)
    - Sterilization via colpotomy: Very obese women, women with an umbilical hernia, or those with a previous umbilical hernia repair
    - Hysterectomy and bilateral oophorectomy: Indicated for severe medical disorders that put the woman at risk with pregnancy
- Male sterilization via vasectomy: Surgically sever and occlude the paired vas deferens; uses local anesthesia; no-scalpel vasectomy freezes scrotal skin; vas tubes are cauterized and occluded through a 4-mm incision

Epidemiology

- 30% of reproductive-age couples choose female sterilization for contraception
- Female sterilization rate is higher in married, divorced, over 30, and African-American women
- Female sterilization: 0.2% (age 15–19) to 47% (age 40–44)
- Male sterilization: 0.2% (age 15–19) to 21% (age 40–44)
- Tubal ligation is the leading contraception in U.S. women over 30

Side Effects

- Tubal occlusion
    - Some pain or discomfort for several days after the operation
    - Post-tubal ligation syndrome (menstrual irregularity and dysmenorrhea) is controversial; most likely due to discontinuing of oral contraceptives
    - Regret (3–25%)
- Conventional vasectomy: Side effects are rare
    - Bleeding and pain/discomfort
    - Scrotal discoloration (for several days)
    - 50% of patients will form antisperm antibodies after the procedure
- No-scalpel vasectomy has less pain and less scrotal discoloration

Alternative Treatments

- Tubal occlusion
    - Mini-laparotomy: Pomeroy method, Irving method, and Uchida method are the most common
    - Laparoscopic: Bipolar electrocoagulation, banding procedures (e.g., Falope Ring Band) and clips (e.g., Hulka-Clemens Clip and the Filshie Clip)
    - Sterilization via colpotomy: Most commonly using the Pomeroy method
    - Hysteroscopic sterilization (Essure permanent birth control procedure) is not yet available in U.S.
- Hysterectomy and bilateral oophorectomy
- OCPs, barrier methods, or intrauterine devices
- Male sterilization
    - Conventional vasectomy (incisional vasectomy) is the most common method in U.S.
    - No-scalpel vasectomy: With or without fascial interposition; with or without open vasectomy

Efficacy

- Tubal occlusion is a highly effective form of permanent sterilization
    - Failure rate of only 0.2–0.4%; failures result from recanalization of the oviduct or tuboperitoneal fistula
    - Irving method: Extremely low failure rate (<0.001)
    - Uchida method: No failures have been reported
    - Highest failure rate was among women age <30 who were sterilized with bipolar coagulation (54.3/1000 procedures) and clip application (52.1/1000 procedures)
- Vasectomy is also highly effective
    - Safer and less expensive than tubal ligation
    - Both conventional vasectomy and no-scalpel vasectomy are equally effective (>99%)
    - Failure rate of only 0.1% (mainly due to beginning intercourse too soon after the procedure)
    - Semen analysis required 1 and 2 months after surgery; two sperm-free ejaculations are proof of sterility

Complications

- Tubal occlusion: Risk of hemorrhage, sepsis, pelvic infection, and fistula formation; risk of death 4/100,000 attributable to anesthesia complications; ectopic pregnancy (7.3/1000 procedures): highest risk with bipolar coagulation; lowest with postpartum partial salpingectomy; gynecologic problems from tubal occlusions necessitating hysterectomy (1.6%); perforation of the uterus, bladder, or bowel with laparoscopy (0.4%)
- Vasectomy complications are rare: Risk of bleeding and infection; sperm granulomas formation at the end of the severed tube; scrotal hematoma; chronic pain syndrome; continued fertility (15–20 ejaculations); higher prostate cancer risk (controversial)

Gynecologic Oncology

ALISON V. CAPE, MD
KAREN M. FREUND, MD, MPH
NEDA LAITEERAPONG
HOPE A. RICCIOTTI, MD
CHRISTINE M. WEEKS, MD

42. Cancer in Pregnancy

Etiology/Pathophysiology

- Cancer is the second most common cause of death for women in their reproductive years; 1 in 1,000 pregnancies are complicated by cancer
- The malignancies most commonly encountered in pregnancy are breast, cervical, melanoma, ovarian, thyroid, leukemia, lymphoma, and colorectal
- Cancer during pregnancy is a therapeutic dilemma—treatment is influenced by ethical, cultural, and religious concerns; the decision to continue pregnancy is made after being informed of the potential risks/benefits
- Chemotherapy during pregnancy is associated with fetal malformations, which correlate highly with the gestational age at the time of exposure
  - Major morphologic abnormalities are most likely between 3 and 8 weeks gestation (organogenesis occurs during this period)
  - Second and third trimester chemotherapy does not appear to carry a significantly increased risk of major fetal anomalies but is associated with low birth weight
- Radiation during the first 20 weeks gestation in doses beyond 200 cGy cause congenital malformations in the majority of fetuses (e.g., microcephaly, retardation); doses in excess of 300 cGy increases the risk of abortion

Differential Dx

- Normal breast changes of pregnancy
- Cervical erosion
- Normal pigmentation changes of pregnancy
- Bleeding in pregnancy
- Normal thyroid enlargement of pregnancy
- Normal hematologic changes of pregnancy
- Hemorrhoids

Presentation

- Note that normal changes of pregnancy may mimic cancer
- Breast cancer: Presents as a painless lump often discovered by the patient
- Cervical cancer: Vaginal bleeding
- Melanoma: An abnormal skin lesion often noted by the patient
- Ovarian cancer: Often found incidentally on prenatal ultrasound; torsion, rupture, hemorrhage
- Thyroid cancer: Thyroid nodules are often palpated at the first prenatal visit
- Leukemia: Hematologic abnormalities, fatigue, fever, infection, easy bleeding, petechiae
- Lymphoma: Enlarged cervical or axillary lymph nodes
- Colorectal cancer: Rectal bleeding, constipation

Diagnosis/Evaluation

- Breast cancer: Breast abnormalities should be evaluated in the same manner as if the patient were not pregnant; however, the increased tissue density of pregnancy makes mammogram interpretation more difficult; fine needle aspiration or excisional biopsy are reliable
- Cervical cancer: If an abnormal Pap smear is found in pregnancy, perform colposcopy with directed biopsies of any areas that are worrisome for invasive cancer; a diagnosis of microinvasion must be followed by a cone biopsy to rule out invasive disease
- Melanoma: Tissue sampling
- Ovarian cancer: Surgical exploration before 18 weeks gestation is acceptable and not associated with fetal wastage
- Thyroid cancer: Biopsy of suspicious nodules
- Leukemia: Hematologic evaluation
- Lymphoma: Biopsy of suspicious nodes
- Colorectal cancer: The majority of colorectal cancers in pregnancy are palpable on rectal examination; endoscopic evaluation is also used

Treatment

- Breast cancer: Excisional biopsy with evaluation of lymph node status as in nonpregnant patients; consider delay of irradiation until after delivery
- Cervical cancer: Deliver fetus by cesarean section, followed by radical hysterectomy; vaginal delivery is reserved for patients with pre-invasive disease or stage Ia
- Melanoma: Surgical excision
- Ovarian cancer: Staging laparotomy
- Thyroid cancer: Total thyroidectomy
- Leukemia: Immediate combination chemotherapy is indicated due to poor prognosis with delay in treatment
- Lymphoma: Chemotherapy for subdiaphragmatic or advanced Hodgkin's disease
- Colorectal cancer: Colon resection with anastomosis may be performed during the first half of pregnancy; in late pregnancy, a diverting colostomy may be necessary

Prognosis/Complications

- Prognoses of breast, cervical, lymphoma, ovarian, and thyroid cancers are not altered by pregnancy
- Breast cancer: Subsequent pregnancies do not adversely affect survival
- Cervical cancer: Complications from cone biopsy in pregnancy are common
- Melanoma: Potential for metastases to fetus
- Ovarian cancer: Torsion/rupture may increase the risk of spontaneous abortion and preterm delivery
- Leukemia: 15% increased risk of stillbirth; 50% increased risk of prematurity; growth restriction
- Lymphoma: Treatment often compromises future reproductive potential
- Colorectal cancer: Delays in diagnosis result in more advanced disease

43. Breast Cancer

Etiology/Pathophysiology

- 211,000 newly diagnosed women in the U.S. per year
- 8% of cases are due to hereditary factors
    - Mutations in BRCA1 or BRCA2 genes are the most common hereditary influences (present in up to 50% of hereditary cases of breast cancer)
- Black women diagnosed with breast cancer have worse prognoses than white women
- Risk factors
    - Increased age
    - Female sex
    - Family history in a first-degree relative, especially if premenopausal
    - Moderate alcohol consumption (3+ drinks/week)
    - Estrogen exposure: Early menarche, late menopause, nulliparity, hormone replacement therapy

Differential Dx

- 90% of breast masses are benign
- Fibrocystic changes
- Fibroadenoma
- Intraductal papilloma
- Breast cysts
- Mastitis or abscess
- Benign lymphadenopathy

Presentation

- Masses suspicious for cancer tend to have distinct characteristics
    - Solitary, discrete, hard, immovable, irregular borders
    - Unilateral masses in breast or axilla
    - Usually nontender, but may be painful
    - Note that benign features of a mass *do not* rule out cancer
- Skin and/or nipple retraction
- Spontaneous bloody nipple discharge
- Erythema suggests inflammatory cancer
- Edema and peau d'orange are signs of advanced cancer
- Paget's disease may present with a scaly lesion of the nipple

Diagnosis/Evaluation

- Clinical breast exam: 11% of breast cancers are missed by mammograms but diagnosed by clinical breast exam
- Mammography is recommended annually in women >40 years
    - Increased density, irregular margins, spiculation, and clustered irregular microcalcifications suggest malignancy
- Ultrasound is used to identify breast cysts and to evaluate lesions that are inconclusive on mammogram
    - Especially useful in young women
- Biopsy with tissue analysis is diagnostic
    - Fine needle aspiration allows for cytology only (i.e., distinguishes malignant from benign cells but may not give tissue diagnosis); most useful in women under age 40 with low-risk lesions
    - Core needle biopsy provides definitive diagnosis; may be also used with imaging for localization and biopsy of non-palpable lesions
    - Excisional biopsy provides definitive diagnosis and may also serve as lumpectomy if entire lesion is removed with adequate margins

Treatment

- Sentinel node and/or axillary node dissection is used for staging in all patients
- Resection of lesion for local therapy
    - 2–5 cm lesions are generally treated by lumpectomy and radiation therapy
    - Lesions >5 cm or multifocal disease are treated with mastectomy
- Systemic treatment is often administered in addition to local resection
    - Hormone therapy (e.g., tamoxifen) is indicated for estrogen/progesterone receptor-positive tumors
    - Chemotherapy is indicated for large tumors (>5 cm), positive lymph nodes, or poor prognostic markers (e.g., positive HER2/neu receptors, inflammatory cancer, poorly differentiated cancers)

Prognosis/Complications

- 5-year survival
    - Ductal carcinoma in situ: 95%
    - Stage I (tumor ≤2 cm): 88%
    - Stage II (tumor 2–5 cm, positive regional lymph nodes): 66%
    - Stage III (tumor ≥5 cm, positive lymph nodes): 36%
    - Stage IV (any metastatic disease): 7%
- Estrogen/progesterone receptor-positive tumors carry a better prognosis
- HER-2/neu receptor-positive tumors are associated with more aggressive disease
- Recurrence may appear up to 10–15 years after diagnosis

44. Solid Ovarian Tumors

Etiology/Pathophysiology

- The classification of ovarian tumors is based on cell of origin
- Epithelial tumors (70%): Serous, mucinous, endometrioid, clear cell, Brenner-transitional cell, mixed mesodermal, and undifferentiated tumors are considered epithelial tumors
- Germ cell tumors (15–20%): Dysgerminoma, endodermal sinus tumor, embryonal carcinoma, polyembryoma, choriocarcinoma, teratoma (dermoid), mixed forms, and gonadoblastoma; germ cell tumors are diseases of young women, with the mean age 19 years; gonadoblastoma and dysgerminoma are often found in patients with gonadal dysgenesis
- Stromal tumors (5–10%): Granulosa stromal cell tumor, Sertoli stromal cell tumor, sex cord tumor with annular tubules, Leydig cell tumor, lipid cell tumor, and gynandroblastoma; usually in postmenopausal women
- Metastatic tumors (5%) most commonly from colon (52%), breast (17%), stomach (10%), and pancreas (10%); Krukenberg tumor is one that metastasizes from stomach and contains pathognomonic "signet-ring cells"
- Age of the patient is extremely important in determining preoperative risk for different types and ordering the appropriate tumor markers

Differential Dx

- Physiologic cysts (follicular, corpus luteum, theca lutein cysts)
- Endometrioma
- Borderline tumors
- Ectopic pregnancy
- Hydrosalpinx or tubo-ovarian abscess, para-ovarian cyst, peritoneal inclusion cyst
- Pedunculated fibroid
- Diverticular/appendiceal abscess
- Fallopian tube cancer (rare)

Presentation

- Palpation of an asymptomatic adnexal mass during pelvic examination
- Vague, ill-defined lower abdominal discomfort, pressure or bloating; abdominal distention; dyspareunia; irregular menstrual cycles
- Precocious puberty with germ cell tumors producing hormones
- Struma ovarii (dermoid) patients can present with hyperthyroidism
- Granulosa cell tumors and thecomas often produce excess estrogen; presentation may include vaginal bleeding, endometrial hyperplasia, or carcinoma
- Sertoli-Leydig cell tumors: 40% of patients show evidence of excess androgen production

Diagnosis/Evaluation

- Physical examination, including a pelvic examination with rectovaginal examination
- Ultrasound: Assessment of size of tumor; evaluation of contralateral ovary; presence of papillations; ascites
- Preoperative evaluation of tumor markers: CA-125 (epithelial tumors, especially serous); AFP (endodermal sinus tumor, embryonal carcinoma); estradiol (granulosa cell tumors, thecomas); LDH (dysgerminoma), hCG (choriocarcinoma, embryonal carcinoma); testosterone (Sertoli cell, Leydig cell tumors)
- Exclusion of extra-ovarian primary, if indicated, through colonoscopy, barium enema, or mammography
- Histologic confirmation, either by laparoscopy or laparotomy, is necessary to establish the diagnosis
- Karyotyping is indicated if a dysgerminoma or gonadoblastoma is suspected to rule out gonadal dysgenesis
- Endometrial biopsy is indicated if there is evidence of excess estrogen production from the tumor

Treatment

- Any solid ovarian tumor requires surgical exploration
- Staging procedure: Laparotomy, peritoneal cavity free fluid/washings for cytology, TAH-BSO, inspection/biopsy intraperitoneal surfaces, biopsies, omentectomy, exploration retroperitoneal spaces, dissect pelvic/para-aortic nodes, debulking in advanced disease
- Surgery that preserves reproductive function may be utilized in young women if frozen section confirms grade 1, stage IA invasive epithelial, borderline, germ cell, and stromal cell tumors
- Gonadoblastoma: Patients with gonadal dysgenesis associated with a Y-chromosome require bilateral gonadectomy to prevent malignant transformation
- Dysgerminomas: Usually stage I and unilateral; biopsy of opposite ovary indicated due to 10–15% bilaterality
- Platinum-based combination chemotherapy is the standard treatment for patients at high risk for recurrence stage I, grade 3; stage IC; and all stage II, III, IV

Prognosis/Complications

- See *Epithelial Ovarian Carcinoma* entry
- Germ cell tumors
  - Dysgerminoma: Survival with early stage disease is >95%; >80% in patients with advanced disease with adjuvant therapy
  - 1–2% of dermoids are malignant teratomas; stage I grade 1 100% survival; 50% for stage III grade 1
  - Endodermal sinus tumor survival rates for patients with stage I or II tumors 60–100%; stage III or IV survival rates 50–75%
- Stromal tumors
  - Granulosa cell is 85–90% stage I; 55–60% with extra-ovarian extension
  - Sertoli-Leydig cell: Poor prognosis with poorly differentiated, otherwise prognosis is good

45. Epithelial Ovarian Carcinoma

Etiology/Pathophysiology

- 1 in 70 women will develop ovarian cancer (median age is 60 years)
- Leading cause of death from gynecologic cancer in the U.S.
- Accounts for 70–85% of all ovarian neoplasms
- Malignant serous tumors are the most common (40%) type; other types include mucinous, endometrioid, clear cell, Brenner-transitional cell, undifferentiated cancer, and mixed mesodermal tumor
- Borderline tumors (tumors of low malignant potential) are epithelial tumors with stratification and increased atypia with intact basement membranes, including serous, mucinous, endometrioid, and clear cell; median age is 39
- Oral contraceptives, term pregnancies, breast-feeding, and tubal ligation *decrease* the risk of developing ovarian cancer
- Associated with three hereditary syndromes: Ovarian cancer syndrome, breast-ovarian cancer syndrome, and hereditary nonpolyposis colorectal cancer syndrome (Lynch syndrome II)
    - –Transmitted as autosomal dominant inheritance with incomplete penetrance
    - –BRCA1 and BRCA2 mutations increase the risk
- There is no effective population-based screening tool for these cancers

Differential Dx

- Physiologic cysts (follicular, corpus luteum, endometrioma, theca lutein cysts)
- Benign ovarian neoplasms
- Ectopic pregnancy
- Hydrosalpinx or tubo-ovarian abscess, para-ovarian cyst, peritoneal inclusion cyst
- Pedunculated fibroids
- Diverticular or appendiceal abscess
- Fallopian tube cancer

Presentation

- Vague, ill-defined lower abdominal discomfort, pressure, or bloating; abdominal distention
- Indigestion; inability to eat normally; nausea; early satiety; constipation
- Low back pain
- Fatigue
- Urinary frequency
- Dyspareunia
- Irregular menstrual cycles
- Precocious puberty (with germ cell tumors that produce hormones)
- Palpation of an asymptomatic adnexal mass during routine pelvic exam

Diagnosis/Evaluation

- Physical examination including pelvic/rectovaginal examination and ultrasound are the most useful diagnostic tools for evaluating the ovary; a pelvic mass on physical exam or ultrasound usually requires surgical exploration
- Ultrasound criteria for surgical exploration: Ovarian cysts >5 cm persistent for 6–8 weeks, solid ovarian tumors, ovarian cysts with papillary vegetations, adnexal mass >10 cm, any tumor with associated ascites, palpable adnexal mass with associated symptoms of torsion or rupture
- Ovarian cancer is a surgical diagnosis and is surgically staged
- CA-125 can be useful tumor marker, but the sensitivity in early disease (stage I) is lower than later stages (in stages II–IV >90% have elevated levels); highest incidence of elevation is in serous histology
- CT/MRI are not helpful in diagnosis, but help to optimize surgical procedures and demonstrate potential metastases
- Colonoscopy, barium enema, mammography may be utilized to exclude an extra-ovarian primary tumor

Treatment

- Staging laparotomy: Peritoneal washings, TAH-BSO, biopsy of peritoneal surfaces/diaphragm, omentectomy, dissection of pelvic and para-aortic nodes, and debulking
    - –Stage IA: Growth limited to one ovary; no ascites or tumor on external surfaces; capsule intact
    - –Stage IB: Growth limited to both ovaries
    - –Stage IC: Tumor on surface of ovaries or capsule ruptured or malignant ascites/peritoneal washings
    - –Stage IIA: Extension to uterus/fallopian tubes
    - –Stage IIB: Extension to pelvic tissues
    - –Stage IIIA: Limited to pelvis with microscopic seeding of abdominal peritoneal surfaces
    - –Stage IIIB: Implants of peritoneal surfaces ≤2 cm
    - –IIIC: Implants >2 cm or retroperitoneal/inguinal nodes
    - –Stage IV: Distant mets or malignant pleural effusion
- Primary cytoreduction with <1.5 cm of residual disease
- Chemotherapy indicated for stages II, III, IV, and some stage I disease

Prognosis/Complications

- Stage IA or B with grade 1 or 2 tumors: 5-year disease-free survival is 91–98%
- Stage I, grade 3; stage IC, II, III, or IV: Platinum-based combination chemotherapy is the standard postoperative treatment; high risk of recurrence; median progression-free survival is 18 months
- Multi-agent chemotherapy is associated with improved disease response rates, enhanced survival times, and improved therapeutic indexes
- Women with hereditary cancer syndromes have a 50% lifetime risk of ovarian cancer; prophylactic oophorectomy after childbearing may be offered

46. Evaluation of an Abnormal Pap Smear

Etiology/Pathophysiology

- More than 3.5 million women in the U.S. each year (7% of Pap smears) have abnormal findings
- Squamous cell carcinoma accounts for 90% of cervical cancers, adenocarcinoma for 10%
    - The main risk factor for squamous cell carcinoma is HPV infection, which is transmitted by sexual contact; condoms are not entirely protective due to scrotal-labial transmission; HPV types 16, 18, 31, 33, 35, and 45 are more likely to have oncogenic potential
    - The main risk factor for adenocarcinoma is DES exposure in utero
- Other epidemiologic factors that may increase the risk of developing abnormal cervical cells include sexual intercourse at an early age, multiple sexual partners, cigarette smoking, STDs (including chlamydia), and immunodeficiency
- Annual Pap smear surveillance is recommended for all women who are sexually active or over 18

Differential Dx

- Postmenopausal cellular alterations (e.g., prominent perinuclear halos, nuclear hyperchromasia, variation in nuclear size, multinucleation)
    - Often misclassified as koilocytotic atypia
- Metaplasia
    - A process whereby the columnar epithelium is replaced by squamous epithelium
    - Appears acetowhite on colposcopy

Presentation

- ASCUS (atypical squamous cells of undetermined significance) may represent reactive or reparative changes secondary to inflammation
- ASC-H (atypical squamous cells, cannot exclude HSIL)
- LSIL (low-grade squamous intra-epithelial lesion or CIN I) is often due to a transient HPV infection
- HSIL (high-grade squamous intra-epithelial lesion or CIN II/III) is associated with viral persistence and higher risk for progression
- AGUS (atypical glandular cells of undetermined significance) has a greater risk of underlying neoplasia
- Squamous cell carcinoma

Diagnosis/Evaluation

- An abnormal Pap smear is not a diagnosis in itself and requires further testing
- ASCUS finding: Repeat Pap smear in 4–6 months
    - Colposcopy is indicated if repeat Pap smear shows ASCUS
    - If a liquid-based Pap smear is used, perform HPV testing on the original liquid-based cytology specimen; all women who test positive for HPV should be referred for colposcopy
    - Colposcopy is recommended for immunosuppressed patients with ASCUS, including all women with HIV
- ASC-H, LSIL, HSIL: Perform colposcopy with directed biopsy
- AGUS: Perform colposcopy with directed biopsies and endocervical curettage to rule out endometrial pathology
- Diagnostic conization should be performed if unsatisfactory colposcopy, uncertainty regarding presence of invasive disease, lesions in endocervical canal, cells on cytologic examination not adequately explained by biopsy specimens, biopsy suggests micro-invasion, or abnormal endocervical glandular cells

Treatment

- Confirmed HSIL cells require excision or destruction to prevent progression to cancer
- Small lesions confined to the exocervix where biopsies have ruled out invasive disease can be destroyed by cryotherapy, laser vaporization, or loop excision
- Larger lesions involving the endocervix must be excised via conization (can be performed as a diagnostic procedure or as a therapeutic procedure) to remove a cone-shaped wedge of the cervix, transformation zone, and all or a portion of the endocervical canal
    - "Cold knife" (or scalpel) conization
    - Loop electrosurgical excision procedure (LEEP): An electrosurgical loop is used to burn through the tissue
    - Laser excision: The laser is used as a knife
- Treatment for a Pap smear confirmed as squamous cell carcinoma may involve conization for small lesions in situ or radical hysterectomy with adjuvant therapy for more extensive disease; see *Cervical Cancer* entry

Prognosis/Complications

- LSIL: The majority of lesions will either spontaneously regress or persist unchanged
- HSIL: The risk of progression to invasive cancer without treatment is 6% by 3 years and as high as 70% by 12 years
- Success rate of cryotherapy, loop excision, and laser ablation are better than 90%
- Cervical surgery is a risk factor for cervical incompetence and cervical stenosis; however, these complications are rare

47. Cervical Cancer

Etiology/Pathophysiology

- Cervical cancer is the second most common cause of cancer-related morbidity and mortality among women in developing countries
- There has been a 75% decrease in the incidence and mortality of cervical cancer in developed countries during the past 50 years secondary to widespread Pap smear screening
- Squamous cell carcinoma accounts for 80% of cervical cancers; adenosquamous accounts for 15%; the remaining cases are rare histologies
- Human papilloma virus is considered the most important factor contributing to the development of cervical intra-epithelial neoplasia (CIN) and cervical cancer; high-risk oncogenic HPV types include 16, 18, 31, 33, 35, and 45
- Major risk factors include early onset of sexual activity, multiple sexual partners, high-risk sexual partner (promiscuous sexual activity, sexual exposure to partner with HPV), and smoking
- Other risk factors include a history of STDs (chlamydia), smoking, high parity, immunosuppression (including HIV), low socioeconomic status, and a previous history of vulvar or vaginal squamous dysplasia

Differential Dx

- Stage 0: Carcinoma in situ
- Stage I: Confined to cervix (Ia microscopic, Ib visible lesions)
- Stage II: Involves vagina but not the lower 1/3; infiltrates parametria but not the sidewall
- Stage III: Involves the lower 1/3 of vagina or extends to pelvic wall; hydronephrosis/nonfunctioning kidney
- Stage IV: Extends beyond pelvis; mucosa of bladder or rectum

Presentation

- Abnormal bleeding (post-coital, intermenstrual, postmenopausal) is the most common initial presentation
- Discharge (may be watery, blood-tinged, mucoid, purulent, or malodorous)
- Classic presentation is intermittent, painless metrorrhagia or spotting that occurs post-coitally or after douching
- As cancer enlarges, bleeding episodes get heavier, more frequent, and longer
- Late signs include referred pain to flank/leg, dysuria, hematuria, rectal bleeding, obstipation, persistent edema of one or both lower extremities, massive hemorrhage, and uremia

Diagnosis/Evaluation

- Cytologic screening followed by colposcopy with directed biopsies; biopsy of gross or palpable lesions
- In cases of suspected microinvasion and early stage cervical cancer, cone biopsy of the cervix is indicated to evaluate the possibility of invasion
- Staging of cervical cancer is by clinical evaluation (not surgical staging as in other gynecologic cancers)
- Staging should include inspection, palpation, colposcopy, endocervical curettage, hysteroscopy, cystoscopy, proctoscopy, intravenous pyelography, and X-ray examination of lungs and skeleton; cone biopsy is considered part of the clinical staging; clinical examination may be performed under anesthesia
- CT and MRI are valuable for treatment planning but are not used for staging; useful for assessing nodal status and extent of tumor within the pelvis
- Laboratory studies include CBC, BUN/creatinine, and liver function tests to evaluate anemia and metastatic disease

Treatment

- Stage 0: Surgical excision, laser ablation, topical 5-FU
- Stage Ia1: Simple hysterectomy
- Ia2 to IIa: Radical hysterectomy and pelvic lymphadenectomy; or whole pelvis radiotherapy
- Stage Ib–IV: Radiation therapy plus cisplatinum-based chemotherapy
- Radical hysterectomy: Removal of uterus, upper 25% vagina, uterosacral/uterovesical ligaments, parametria, pelvic lymph node dissection
- Adjuvant postoperative radiation with intermediate/high-risk factors for recurrent disease
  - High risk: + or close resection margins, + lymph nodes, microscopic parametrial involvement
  - Intermediate risk: Large tumor size, deep cervical stromal invasion, lymphovascular space invasion
- Primary radiation therapy consists of external beam radiation plus brachytherapy to increase radiation dose delivery to the primary central tumor

Prognosis/Complications

- 5-year survival

–Stage I:	Squamous	65–90%
	Adenocarcinoma	70–75%
–Stage II:	Squamous	45–80%
	Adenocarcinoma	30–40%
–Stage III:	Squamous	up to 60%
	Adenocarcinoma	20–30%
–Stage IV:	Squamous	<15%
	Adenocarcinoma	<15%

- Lymph node status is the most important prognostic factor after stage
- Radical hysterectomy leaves the vagina in more functional condition than radiation; radiation therapy results in a reduction in length, caliber, and lubrication of the vagina; ovarian function can be preserved with surgery in young women

48. Uterine Cancer

Etiology/Pathophysiology

- Uterine cancers include endometrial cancer and uterine sarcoma
- Endometrial cancer is the most common malignancy of the female genital tract and the fourth most common malignancy in women (after breast, lung, colon); median age of onset is 61; however, 20–25% are premenopausal
- Types of endometrial carcinoma include adenocarcinoma (80%), mucinous (5%), clear cell (5%), papillary serous (4%), and squamous (1%)
- Two pathogenic types of endometrial cancer
  - Type I: Estrogen-related; associated with hyperplasia; presents as low-grade endometrioid tumor; risk factors include obesity, chronic anovulation, late menopause, nulliparity, hypertension, cancer of breast/ovary, and diabetes
  - Type II: Appears unrelated to estrogen/hyperplasia; tends to present with higher grade tumors of poor prognostic types (papillary serous, clear cell)
- There is an excess risk for endometrial cancer with unopposed estrogen, which is reduced/eliminated by concurrent progestin therapy; tamoxifen results in a two- to -three-fold increased risk of endometrial cancer; however, benefits in breast cancer risk reduction are thought to outweigh this risk
- Uterine sarcoma: Rare, 3–5% of all uterine cancers; poor prognosis; arises from glands and myometrium; primarily in women 40–60

Differential Dx

- IA: limited to endometrium; IB invades <1/2 myometrium; IC >1/2 myometrium
- IIA endocervical glandular involvement; IIB stromal invasion
- IIIA uterine serosa or malignant cells in peritoneal fluid; IIIB vaginal involvement; IIIC pelvic/ para-aortic lymph nodes
- IVA invasion of bladder/bowel mucosa; IVB distant metastasis

Presentation

- Endometrial cancer
  - 90% of patients present with abnormal uterine bleeding
  - Pelvic pressure/pain
  - Prolonged/heavy periods, intermenstrual spotting
  - Pyometria and hematometria
  - Endometrial cells on Pap smear out of phase with menstrual cycle or in a postmenopausal woman
- Uterine sarcoma
  - Abdominal mass/pain
  - Rapidly enlarging uterus

Diagnosis/Evaluation

- Physical examination, including pelvic examination/Pap smear
- Endometrial biopsy can make a definitive diagnosis and spare patient the need for hospitalization and anesthesia
- Hysteroscopy and D & C may be indicated if an endometrial biopsy cannot be performed due to patient discomfort, cervical stenosis, or insufficient tissue
- Ultrasound is indicated, if endometrial stripe thickness is <5 mm hyperplasia or carcinoma is unlikely
- Postmenopausal women with uterine bleeding should be evaluated for endometrial cancer; 20% will have a genital malignancy
- Uterine cancer is surgically staged
- Laboratory studies include CBC, BUN/creatinine, and liver function tests (preoperative and metastatic disease evaluation)
- Metastatic workup includes chest X-ray, CT, sigmoidoscopy/ barium enema (for patients with palpable disease outside uterus or bowel symptoms); include brain, liver, and bone scans only if evidence of distant disease

Treatment

- Endometrial Cancer
  - Surgical treatment: Total abdominal hysterectomy with bilateral salpingo-oopherectomy; peritoneal washings for cytologic evaluation
  - The decision to perform lymph node sampling depends on the depth of myometrial invasion; if >1/2 myometrial invasion, pelvic/para-aortic lymphadenectomy is indicated at the time of initial surgery due to the risk for lymph node involvement
  - Postoperative radiation decreases the risk of recurrence if ≥ stage IC or grade 3
  - High-dose progestin therapy may be used for advanced or recurrent disease
- Uterine sarcoma
  - Total abdominal hysterectomy with bilateral salpingo-oopherectomy with or without adjuvant radiation

Prognosis/Complications

- Endometrial cancer 5-year survival
  - Stage I   90%
  - Stage II   75%
  - Stage III   40%
  - Stage IV   10%
  - Histologic grade is the most important prognostic factor; depth of invasion is the second most important prognostic factor; adenosquamous, clear cell, and papillary serous carcinomas have worse prognoses than adenocarcinoma
- Uterine sarcoma has a poor prognosis
  - The most important prognostic factor is surgical stage
  - 5-year survival at stage I is 50%; metastases 20%

49. Vaginal Cancer

Etiology/Pathophysiology

- Only 1–2% of genital tract cancers originate in the vaginal tissues
- Squamous cell carcinoma accounts for approximately 90% of primary vaginal cancers
    - Patient age ranges from 30–90 years
    - The average age at diagnosis is approximately 60 years
- Vaginal intra-epithelial neoplasia (VIN) is considered a premalignant lesion, analogous to cervical in situ lesions; however, there is less information regarding the magnitude of premalignant potential, transition times, and factors influencing the transition than in cervical lesions
- Other types of primary vaginal cancers include adenocarcinoma, melanoma, sarcoma, and endodermal sinus tumors
- Most malignant vaginal lesions are secondary, occurring as extensions of cervical or vulvar carcinoma, or as metastatic cancers that usually arise in the bladder, rectum, uterus, or ovary

Differential Dx

- Squamous cell carcinoma
- Melanoma
- Sarcoma
- Adenocarcinoma
- Endodermal sinus tumor
- Metastasis or extension of other tumors
- Vaginal intra-epithelial neoplasia
- Vaginal polyps
- Vaginal ulcers

Presentation

- VIN usually presents as an abnormal Pap smear; usually asymptomatic, but may have post-coital staining or vaginal discharge; a mucosal lesion may be detected on physical exam
- Vaginal cancer
    - Abnormal bleeding or blood-tinged discharge
    - Bleeding with intercourse
    - Anterior wall lesions may cause urinary symptoms (e.g., frequency, dysuria, hematuria)
    - Rectal involvement may manifest as tenesmus, melena, or pain
    - Many patients have no symptoms, with the diagnosis found incidentally on pelvic exam or in response to abnormal cytologic smear findings

Diagnosis/Evaluation

- Vaginal cancer: Lesions vary and may appear as exophytic growths, superficial plaques, or ulcers; diagnosis is confirmed by a biopsy that shows neoplastic epidermoid cells invading the submucosal tissues and the vascular and lymphatic spaces
- Staging is based on history and clinical exam; in addition, chest X-ray, intravenous pyelogram, barium enema, cystoscopy, and proctosigmoidoscopy are performed to determine local or distant spread
    - 0 = in situ
    - I = limited to vaginal wall
    - II = involving subvaginal tissue but not pelvic wall
    - III = extending to the pelvic wall
    - IV = extending beyond the true pelvis or involving the mucosa of the bladder or rectum
- Diagnosis of VIN is established by colposcopically-directed biopsies of the vagina; lesions tend to be multifocal, usually in the upper third of the vagina; colposcopic findings include epithelium that turns white with acetic acid, and blood vessel patterns exhibiting punctation and mosaicism

Treatment

- VIN: Therapeutic options include surgical excision, chemotherapy, or laser ablation
    - Surgical: Wide local excision with primary repair for isolated lesions; total vaginectomy if widespread
    - Chemotherapy with topical 5-FU: Carries the advantage of treating the entire epithelial surface at risk from this potentially multifocal disease
    - Carbon dioxide laser ablation: Has the advantage of specifically targeting treatment to diseased areas in multifocal disease
- Vaginal cancer: Radiation treatment is the primary therapy for vaginal squamous cell carcinoma; however, in some patients, surgery is an option
    - Radiation uses a combined approach of external radiation therapy and local implants
    - Surgical excision as primary therapy applies only to small, localized tumors located in the upper third of the vagina

Prognosis/Complications

- Vaginal intra-epithelial neoplasia has 80% remission rate with treatment
- Topical 5-FU side effects include pain, vulvar irritation, and dysuria
- Prognosis for vaginal squamous cell carcinoma depends primarily on the extent of disease
    - Overall 5-year survival rate is 45%
    - Stage I disease treated with radiation therapy results in 5-year survival rates of 80–90%
    - Stage II disease has 45–58% 5-year survival
    - Stage III disease has 25–40% 5-year survival
    - Stage IV disease has 10% 5-year survival

50. Vulvar Cancer

Etiology/Pathophysiology

- Malignant neoplasms of the vulva represent 5% of malignancies of the female genital tract
- 90% are squamous cell carcinoma
- The vulva may develop skin malignancies, including adenocarcinoma, sarcoma, verrucous, melanoma, basal cell carcinoma, and Paget's disease
- Risk factors for the development of squamous carcinoma include chronic inflammatory diseases of the vulva (such as some vulvar dystrophies), poor hygiene, and age >70 years; risk factors associated with cervical cancer (e.g., number of sexual partners, abnormal Pap smear, HPV, smoking, immunosuppresion) also increase the risk for vulvar cancer
- Vulvar intra-epithelial neoplasia is associated with HPV 16, and to a lesser extent HPV 18 and 31; it is often multifocal, and may occur in conjunction with vaginal and cervical squamous neoplasias; immunosuppression and cigarette smoking are risks for progression to invasive disease
- Vulvar intra-epithelial neoplasia is diagnosed more commonly today, and it is appearing in younger women; the mean age of invasive vulvar carcinoma has remained stable (early 60s); the mean age of patients with vulvar carcinoma in situ has dropped from 53 to 42 years in the past 30 years

Differential Dx

- Folliculitis
- Condyloma acuminatum
- Mycotic vulvitis
- Chancroid
- Molluscum contagiosum
- Psoriasis
- Seborrheic dermatitis
- Lichen planus
- Lichen sclerosis
- Bartholin's duct cyst/absess
- Lipoma
- Hydradenoma
- Trauma

Presentation

- Vulvar lesion noted by patient; pruritus, bleeding, growth of a lesion
- May be an incidental finding on examination; 20% of patients with vulvar intra-epithelial neoplasia have no symptoms
- Diagnoses of vulvar disease are often delayed because of patient embarrassment in seeking treatment
- Paget's disease is characterized by red raised lesions that are often dotted with pale white islands of epithelium; lesions may occur at any site on the vulva or perineum
- Melanoma: Most lesions involve the clitoris and labia minora; usually noticed by the patient because of enlargement of a pre-existing mole or because of bleeding or pruritus

Diagnosis/Evaluation

- Any persistent lesion should be evaluated for neoplasia; there is little correlation between appearance and histopathology of a vulvar lesion
- The diagnosis of vulvar intra-epithelial neoplasia is made by directed biopsy; vulvar colposcopy after a 5-minute soak with 5% acetic acid can be helpful; a punch biopsy device is ideal for directed vulvar biopsies; careful inspection of the vulva during the pelvic examination is required to detect the sometimes subtle color changes associated with this disease
- Vulvar cancer is surgically staged: Stage 0 = carcinoma in situ; Stage I = tumor confined to the vulva or perineum; ≤2 cm, nodes are not palpable; Stage II = tumor confined to the vulva or perineum; >2 cm, nodes are not palpable; Stage III = tumor of any size with adjacent spread to the lower urethra, vagina, anus, and/or unilateral regional lymph node metastasis; Stage IVA = tumor invades upper urethra, bladder mucosa, rectal mucosa, or pelvic bone with or without bilateral regional node metastasis; Stage IVB = any distant metastasis, including pelvic lymph nodes

Treatment

- Vulvar intra-epithelial neoplasia: Therapy is surgical, either excisional or ablative; laser vaporization is an ideal treatment because it allows for highly tailored treatment with minimal scar formation
- Vulvar squamous cell carcinoma
  - <2 cm lesions: Radical wide local excision with ipsilateral groin node dissection; if a positive node is detected at the time of frozen section of the ipsilateral nodes, the contralateral inguinal nodes are explored
  - Early, but centrally located, lesions: 3-incision radical vulvectomy is preferred; if surgical margins on the vulva are within 1 cm, or ≥2 inguinal nodes are positive, adjuvant radiotherapy to the vulva, pelvic nodes, or inguinal nodes may be required
  - Advanced vulvar lesions involving the urethra, anal sphincter, or vagina: A primary surgical approach would involve an extensive resection or possible exenteration; an alternative is radiotherapy and/or chemotherapy

Prognosis/Complications

- Laser vaporization for vulvar intra-epithelial neoplasia: There is substantial pain after surgery and care of the surgical sites is critical to prevent secondary infections
- 5-year survival rates for carcinoma of the vulva: Stage I, 94%; stage II, 89%; stage III, 71%; stage IV, 19%
- 5-year survival rates for vulvar melanoma range from 8–55%; survival data are based on the depth of penetration
- Vulvar Paget's disease is associated with underlying carcinoma 25% of the time; there may be a co-existing underlying adenocarcinoma of the vulva; carcinoma may develop distant from the site of the intra-epithelial lesion, such as carcinoma of the breast, cervix, colon, or skin

51. Gestational Trophoblastic Neoplasia

Etiology/Pathophysiology

- Gestational trophoblastic neoplasia (GTN) is associated with unregulated trophoblastic proliferation/invasion
  - Benign GTN includes complete and partial molar pregnancy
  - Malignant GTN includes invasive mole, choriocarcinoma, and placental site trophoblastic tumor; molar pregnancy may precede malignant disease (50%), but it may be preceded by any gestation
- Etiology is unknown; complete moles have 46, XX karyotype, with all chromosomes of paternal origin; partial moles have triploid karyotype with the extra set of chromosomes of paternal origin; possible etiology includes genetic abnormalities in fertilization, differentiation, pronuclear cleavage, implantation, myometrial invasion, and host immunologic tolerance
- Increased incidence in young or old women (<15 or >40 years) and Asians
- Risk factors for development of malignant GTN include delayed hemorrhage after molar evacuation (75%); theca lutein cyst >5cm (60%); acute pulmonary insufficiency (58%); uterus large for dates (45%); hCG >100,000 (45%); second molar gestation (40%); and maternal age >40 years (25%)
- GTN is highly curable, as it is extremely sensitive to chemotherapy; it produces the tumor marker hCG, making it simple to track the disease

Differential Dx

- Stage I: Confined to the uterine corpus
- Stage II: Outside uterus but confined to pelvis and vagina
- Stage III: Pulmonary metastasis
- Stage IV: Distant metastasis to brain, liver, kidneys, or GI tract

Presentation

- Vaginal bleeding in the first trimester
- Uterine size greater than expected
- Nausea/vomiting; hyperemesis
- Vaginal passage of vesicular tissue
- Pre-eclampsia in the first trimester is almost pathognomonic
- Hyperthyroidism from production of thyrotropin-like compound
- Acute respiratory distress due to trophoblastic pulmonary embolization
- Theca lutein cysts of the ovary
- Metastatic disease: Trophoblastic tumors are perfused with fragile vessels; thus, bleeding may occur from metastatic sites, including lung (80%), vagina (30%), brain (10%), and liver (10%); symptoms include hemoptysis and neurologic deficits

Diagnosis/Evaluation

- Careful history and physical exam, including pelvic exam
- Ultrasound findings include multiple echoes formed by the interface of molar villi and surrounding tissue; patients with lung (seen on chest X-ray) or vaginal metastasis should be evaluated for liver/brain metastasis via CT scans
- Patients with partial moles usually do not have excessive uterine size, theca lutein cysts, pre-eclampsia, hyperthyroidism, or respiratory problems; thus, the clinical diagnosis is often a missed abortion; however, pathologic evaluation of the products of conception reveals the diagnosis
- Laboratory studies include β-hCG, CBC, electrolytes, BUN/creatinine, liver and thyroid function tests
- Pathology: Partial moles have focal swelling and trophoblastic hyperplasia, with fetal tissue often present; complete moles contain no fetal tissue; chorionic villi have generalized swelling and hyperplasia; persistent GTN may have features of molar tissue or choriocarcinoma (sheets of anaplastic cytotrophoblast and syncytiotrophoblast)

Treatment

- Molar pregnancy: Evacuate uterus via suction curettage followed by sharp curettage to remove residual tissue
  - Rh-negative women should receive Rh-immune globulin
  - Follow-up β-hCG determinations to ensure remission (1–2 week intervals until two negative levels, then monthly levels for 6 months; be sure to use a reliable contraceptive method during this time, such as OCPs)
- Persistent GTN
  - Initial treatment is single agent chemotherapy or hysterectomy with adjunctive chemotherapy
  - Resistant disease is treated with combination chemotherapy or hysterectomy with adjunctive chemotherapy; local resection
  - Stage IV disease is treated with intensive combination chemotherapy, selective radiation, and surgery
  - Follow up with weekly hCG levels until normal 3x; then monthly until normal 12x; patients require 12 consecutive months of contraception

Prognosis/Complications

- After treatment with chemotherapy, most patients can expect normal reproductive outcomes in future pregnancies
- Risk of persistent GTN after partial mole is 0–11%; after complete mole risk of uterine invasion is 15% and metastasis 4%
- Metastatic GTN remission rate: Stage I–III disease: 80–99%; stage IV disease: 77%
- Good prognosis metastatic GTN (58% remission) has none of following: Brain/liver metastases; serum hCG >40,000 mIU/mL; previous chemotherapy; symptoms (antecedent pregnancy) >4 months
- Poor prognosis metastatic GTN (38% remission) includes disease previously treated with chemotherapy; liver metastases; or brain metastasis

Common Non-Gynecologic Medical Issues in Women

ALEXANDRA BAGERIS
PHYLLIS L. CARR, MD
CYNTHIA H. CHUANG, MD
DONNA COHEN, MD
MICHELE DAVID, MD, MPH, MBA
MATTHEW FREIBERG, MD
KAREN M. FREUND, MD, MPH
NEDA LAITEERAPONG
OMAR MULLA-OSSMAN, MD
DANIEL P. NEWMAN, MD
MARY ELLEN PAVONE, MD
MARION P. RUSSELL, MD
MICHELE SINOPOLI, MD
JILL WOODS-CLAY, MD

52. Urinary Tract Infections

Etiology/Pathophysiology

- Infection of the lower (cystitis) and/or upper (pyelonephritis) urinary tract
- 50% of adult women report a UTI at some point during their lives
- Uncomplicated UTIs are generally due to *E. coli* (80%) or *Staphylococcus saprophyticus* (20%)
    - Commonly associated with sexual intercourse (especially with spermicide containing contraceptive, and diaphragm use)
- Complicated UTIs are often due to antibiotic resistant organisms, including *E. coli, Pseudomonas, Proteus, Klebsiella, S. aureus, Enterococcus, Serratia,* and *Enterobacter*
    - Predisposing factors for complicated UTIs include age, hospital-acquired infection, indwelling catheter, urinary tract instrumentation, pregnancy, anatomic abnormality, neurogenic bladder, diabetes, immunosuppression
    - May result in systemic illness, bacteremia, and/or treatment failure
- Most cases of pyelonephritis are due to ascending bacteria from the lower urinary tract; however, hematogenous spread may play a role in some cases (e.g., renal parenchymal abscess in an IV drug user)
    - May be associated with renal and collecting system anomalies, renal stones, neurogenic bladder (diabetes or spinal cord injury), underlying renal disease

Differential Dx

- Urethritis
- Vaginitis
- Cervicitis
- Pelvic inflammatory disease
- Chlamydia
- Gonorrhea

Presentation

- Dysuria
- Urinary frequency
- Urinary urgency
- Suprapubic pain/tenderness
- Hematuria may be present
- Pyelonephritis will additionally present with fever (may be high-grade and persistent even with appropriate antibiotic therapy), nausea, vomiting, flank pain, and CVA tenderness
- Elderly may present with mental status change, fever, abdominal pain, or without symptoms

Diagnosis/Evaluation

- Directed history and physical examination, including temperature, abdominal examination, and assessment of costovertebral angle for tenderness
- Empiric therapy without further workup (based on presentation alone) is acceptable in women with recurrent acute uncomplicated cystitis
- Urinalysis showing pyuria and hematuria suggests UTI
    - Bacteriuria is not required for a diagnosis of acute uncomplicated cystitis as there are low pathogen quantities
- Urine dipstick is generally considered positive if leukocyte esterase (detects pyuria) or nitrites (detects *Enterobacter,* which converts urinary nitrate to nitrite) are present
- Urine culture should be performed in all pregnant, immunocompromised, and diabetic women
- If pyelonephritis is suspected, CBC with differential and creatinine for renal function are indicated
- Renal ultrasound or CT are indicated in pyelonephritis that is refractory to treatment (rule out abscess, obstruction, or stone)

Treatment

- Antibiotic choice depends on local drug resistance (e.g., in some regions, 35% of *E. coli* resistant to trimethoprim/sulfamethoxazole)
- Acute uncomplicated cystitis: 3-day course of trimethoprim/sulfamethoxazole or a fluoroquinolone
    - Pregnant women should be treated with a 3–7 day course of amoxicillin, nitrofurantoin, or cephalexin
- Acute complicated cystitis: 7–14 day course of a fluoroquinolone is sufficient in most cases
    - Parenteral therapy (levofloxacin, ceftriaxone, or aminoglycoside) is indicated for multidrug resistance or allergy to fluoroquinolones
    - Ampicillin or amoxicillin should be added if gram-positive cocci (e.g., *Staphylococcus*) are present
- Daily or post-coital prophylaxis for frequent recurrences
- Uncomplicated pyelo: 10–14 days of oral fluoroquinolone
- Complicated pyelo: 14 day course of IV fluoroquinolone, ampicillin plus gentamicin, or penicillin/antipenicillinase

Prognosis/Complications

- If symptoms re-occur soon after treatment, re-evaluation of diagnosis with pelvic examination should be considered
- No long-term adverse effects on renal function or mortality are associated with acute cystitis in young healthy adult women, even with frequent recurrences
- Acute uncomplicated cystitis does not require routine follow up
- Acute complicated cystitis requires follow up with urine culture only if symptomatic
- Pregnant women require follow-up urine cultures 1–2 weeks post-treatment
- Urology referral may be necessary for cases of recurrent pyelonephritis or any case that remains symptomatic after 72 hours of therapy

53. Upper Respiratory Tract Infections

Etiology/Pathophysiology

- Upper respiratory infections (URIs) include a variety of illnesses including sinusitis, rhinitis, laryngitis, pharyngitis, and epiglottitis
- The common cold is the most common URI
- More than 50% have a viral etiology; other causes include bacterial infection, anatomic deformities (deviated septum, nasal polyps), allergy, dental disease
- 0.5–2% viral URIs become secondarily infected with bacteria
- Families of common viral pathogens include rhinovirus, para-influenza virus, influenza viruses, coronavirus, adenovirus, less commonly EBV, CMV, HIV
- Common bacterial pathogens include *Streptococcus pneumoniae*, *Haemophilus influenzae*, and *Moraxella catarrhalis*; group A streptococcus, group C streptococcus, mixed anaerobic infections, diphtheria
- Sinusitis is an inflammation of the paranasal sinuses
    - Impaired drainage of the sinus ostiae
    - Chronic infection is usually bacterial (*S. pneumoniae*, *H. influenzae*, *M. catarrhalis*)
- Streptococcal pharyngitis (strep throat): Group A β-hemolytic streptococcal infection of pharynx (30% of bacterial pharyngitis)

Differential Dx

- Common cold
- Influenza
- CMV
- EBV
- Mumps
- Rubeola
- Epiglottitis
- Bronchitis
- Atypical pneumonia
- Strep throat
- Allergic rhinitis

Presentation

- Sneezing
- Non-productive cough
- Malaise
- Sinus pain
- Mucopurulent nasal discharge
- Headache
- Maxillary toothache
- Mild lymphadenopathy
- Low-grade fever

Diagnosis/Evaluation

- Usually a clinical diagnosis
- Throat culture to rule out strep pharyngitis
- CBC if symptoms persist or high fever
- Sinus radiographs or CT for chronic sinusitis refractory to antibiotic therapy
- EBV and CMV titers if suspected
- The challenge is differentiating between viral and bacterial infections. Features suggesting bacterial infection, especially after a course of 5 or more days
    - Mucopurulent nasal discharge
    - Productive cough
    - Bacterial sinusitis generally has symptoms that worsen after 5 days and persist longer than 10 days
    - Pharyngeal exudates, fever >37.7°C (100°F) and marked lymphadenopathy suggest bacterial infection (strep)

Treatment

- Symptomatic therapy is often sufficient, as most infections are of viral origin (even if fever and productive cough are present)
- Common cold: Rest, fluids, and acetaminophen; humidification of inspired air; decongestants, 2–3 days of Afrin nasal spray, nasal steroids, or atropine
- Strep pharyngitis: Penicillin V 250 mg QID for 10 days (erythromycin 350 mg TID for 10 days for penicillin-allergic patients)
- Sinusitis: 10-day course of amoxicillin, a cephalosporin or erythromycin if allergic to penicillin; shorter courses have recently been successful; fluoroquinolones if resistance is suspected; in pregnancy, longer duration of treatment is frequently needed secondary to general swelling of the mucous membranes; fluoroquinolones are not recommended, as studies in animals show irreversible drug-induced arthropathy (joint disease); there is no clear evidence of birth defects in humans

Prognosis/Complications

- Expected course is 6–10 days; course can be prolonged in pregnancy secondary to general swelling of mucous membranes resulting in more severe bronchitis and sinusitis
- Complications of viral URI include lower respiratory tract infection, rhinitis medicamentosa, and otitis media
- Complications of strep pharyngitis include rheumatic fever, post-streptococcal glomerulonephritis, and peritonsillar abscess

54. Lower Respiratory Tract Infections

Etiology/Pathophysiology

- "Typical" pneumonia: *Streptococcus pneumoniae, Haemophilus influenzae, Staphylococcus aureus,* gram negatives (e.g., *Pseudomonas*)
- "Atypical" pneumonia: *Chlamydia, Legionella,* and *Mycoplasma,* viral etiologies (e.g., RSV, influenza, HIV, CMV, SARS)
- Aspiration pneumonia: Gram negatives and anaerobes from oral flora
- Other causes are associated with disease states (e.g., HIV), include *Pneumocystis carinii, Cryptococcus, Nocardia,* and *Mycobacterium*
- Incidence: 20 million cases annually
- 20% of cases result in hospitalization
- Risk factors include smoking, asthma, immunosuppression (e.g., diabetes, HIV), glucocorticoid therapy, hypogammaglobulinemia, post-splenectomy
- Most bacterial pneumonias in pregnant women occur in smokers and are caused by *S. pneumoniae*; there has also been a resurgence of pneumonia due to influenza; routine use of influenza vaccine is recommended after 13 weeks gestation to prevent the complications of influenza in pregnancy

Differential Dx

- Chemical pneumonitis
- Pulmonary edema
- Lung cancer
- Hemorrhage
- COPD
- Bronchitis
- Upper respiratory infection
- Pulmonary embolus
- Bronchiectasis
- Tuberculosis

Presentation

- "Typical" pneumonia
  - Cough (90%)
  - Purulent sputum
  - Fevers
  - Rigors/chills (15–40%)
  - Pleuritic chest pain (30%)
- "Atypical" pneumonia constitutes 20–40% of all pneumonias
  - Historically presents with subclinical symptoms—"walking pneumonia"
  - Dry cough
  - Gradual onset
  - However, may present with any of the above symptoms and result in fulminant life-threatening infection
- Extrapulmonary symptoms include nausea, vomiting, diarrhea, myalgias, and headache

Diagnosis/Evaluation

- Physical exam may reveal localized crackles/rales
- Laboratory studies include CBC (leukocytosis); the presence of leukopenia indicates a poorer prognosis
- Chest X-ray is the gold standard for diagnosis
  - Lobar pneumonia indicates a localized area of opacification
  - Interstitial pneumonia
  - Chest X-ray cannot delineate "atypical" from "typical" disease
- Blood cultures are positive in only 30% of patients
- Serologic testing is indicated if an atypical organism is suspected; however, these tests often take time and treatment should never be withheld while awaiting results
- Sputum culture and Gram stain may help broaden therapy but is often unsatisfactory (need >25 PMNs and <10 epithelial cells/HPF)
- A pathogen is found in only 60% of patients
- Calculate the pneumonia severity index

Treatment

- Treatment is determined by the severity of illness
- There are separate guidelines produced by the Infectious Disease Society of America, the American Thoracic Society, and the British Thoracic Society
- General recommendations
  - Outpatient therapy with macrolide alone
  - Inpatient therapy with a β-lactam (e.g., third-generation cephalosporin) +/– macrolide (e.g., clarithromycin)
  - Severe disease or ICU: β-lactam + quinolone or macrolide
- Patients should be treated for 10–14 days (except for azithromycin: 3–5 days)
- Quinolones should be reserved for hospitalized patients who are severely ill or penicillin-allergic
- If concern for pseudomonal infection, begin empiric coverage with double treatment (e.g., anti-pseudomonal β-lactam and fluoroquinolone +/– gentamicin)

Prognosis/Complications

- Hospitalization rate: 20–25%
- Mortality
  - Outpatient 1%
  - Inpatient may approach 25%
  - Sixth leading cause of death
  - Increased risk factors for mortality: Age >65, other underlying disease such as DM, HIV, COPD, male gender, respirations >30, hypoxia, hypothermia, hypotension; Infection with *S. pneumoniae, S. aureus, Legionella*
- Loss of work is typically 15 days
- Complications include lung abscess, necrotizing pneumonia (often from aspiration of oral anaerobes), empyema, and purulent pleural effusion

55. Asthma

Etiology/Pathophysiology

- Asthma is defined as a reversible (completely or partially) airway obstruction
  - Inflammatory cells result in airway swelling and edema
  - Increased airway smooth muscle responsiveness secondary to inflammation
  - It is thought that the airway swelling is the major factor causing obstruction
- Prevalence is increased in developed nations, with increasing prevalence in the U.S.
- Death rate is also increasing
  - Blacks and minorities have increased death rates compared to whites
- Affects all ages
- There is increased risk for males in childhood and for women over 40
- Asthma is the most common obstructive pulmonary disease in pregnancy (0.4–1.3% of women)

Differential Dx

- COPD
- Pulmonary edema
- Pulmonary embolus
- Bronchiectasis
- Posterior nasal drip syndrome
- Gastroesophageal reflux disease
- Sarcoidosis
- Upper airway obstruction
- Churg-Strauss vasculitis

Presentation

- Classic triad of cough, wheezing, and dyspnea
  - The more of the above present, the more likely the diagnosis
- May also be exposure-induced (e.g., following exercise, cold air exposure, aspirin ingestion)
- Chest pain may be present
- Cough-variant asthma

Diagnosis/Evaluation

- Note history of exposure to known allergens or triggers, frequency of symptoms, and presence of nighttime symptoms
- Exam may reveal high-pitched musical wheezes, increased ratio of inspiration to expiration (I:E ratio >1:2), pulsus paradoxus, decreased oxygen saturation, use of accessory muscles for respiration, and inability to speak in full sentences
- Pulmonary function tests are the key to diagnosis
- Peak flow meter is useful for patients on daily meds to monitor disease, but results vary widely among patients
- Spirometry: Measure FEV_1/FVC to determine obstruction
- If spirometry is normal, check response to a β_2 agonist or methacholine challenge
- Consider allergen skin testing
- Classification of severity is based on symptom frequency
  - Mild intermittent: <2 days/wk, <2 nights/mo, PF >80%
  - Mild persistent: 3–6 days/wk, 3–4 nights/mo, PF >80%
  - Moderate persistent: Daily, >1 night/week, PF 61–79%
  - Severe persistent: Continuous day symptoms, frequent night symptoms, and PF/FEV_1 <60%

Treatment

- Treatment is determined by severity
- All patients are treated with a short-acting β_2 agonist (albuterol)
- Mild intermittent: Short-acting β_2 agonist PRN only
- Mild persistent: Add a low-dose inhaled steroid (second-line therapies are leukotriene antagonists, cromolyn sodium, or theophylline)
- Moderate persistent: Low/medium-dose inhaled steroids, second-line agents, plus a long-acting β_2 agonist (salbuterol)
- Severe persistent: High-dose inhaled steroids plus a long-acting β_2 agonist; may require oral steroids
- Acute exacerbations are often treated with an oral steroid taper over weeks or a short burst over days
- Administer a yearly influenza immunization, which is safe in pregnancy

Prognosis/Complications

- Death rates from asthma are increasing
- Respiratory failure may require intubation
- Status asthmaticus: Inability to reverse bronchospasm with therapy
- Long-term systemic steroid complications include adrenal suppression and osteoporosis (inhaled steroids may result in a small decrease in bone mineral density)
- Asthma in pregnancy
  - 49% of patients have no change in asthma severity; 29% improve; 22% worsen
  - No change in peak flow or FEV_1
  - Aggressive treatment of symptoms to prevent hypoxia
  - β_2 agonists and steroids are considered to be safe in pregnancy; theophylline has been proven safe; data on leukotriene antagonists are not yet available

56. Thyroid Disease

Etiology/Pathophysiology

- Hyperthyroidism is a clinical state that affects 2% of women and results from excess of circulating thyroid hormone
  - Graves' disease: Stimulation of thyroid TSH receptors by immunoglobulins
  - Toxic multinodular goiter: Nodules insidious, usually benign; occurs in middle-aged and elderly patients
  - Toxic adenoma: Solitary autonomously functioning nodule; usually benign
- Hypothyroidism is a clinical state resulting from inadequate secretion of thyroid hormone; incidence increases with age (6% of women >60 years)
- Primary hypothyroidism causes >90% of cases
  - Hashimoto's thyroiditis is the most common cause: Immune-mediated destruction of TSH receptors, microsomal enzymes, and glandular antigens
  - Prior treatment of hyperthyroidism with radio-iodine or subtotal thyroidectomy
  - Postpartum thyroiditis: A variant of Hashimoto's disease; peaks 3–4 months postpartum
- Secondary hypothyroidism results from a pituitary process that leads to a deficiency of TSH

Differential Dx

- Hyperthyroidism
  - Anxiety
  - Diabetes mellitus
  - Malignancy
  - Pheochromocytoma
  - Perimenopausal state
- Hypothyroidism
  - Depression
  - Dementia
  - Nephrotic syndrome
  - CHF
  - Primary amyloidosis

Presentation

- Hyperthyroidism
  - Anxiety/emotional lability
  - Increased perspiration
  - Heat intolerance
  - Palpitations/tachycardia
  - Tremor
  - Weakness
  - Weight loss (despite appetite)
  - Oligomenorrhea/amenorrhea
- Hypothyroidism
  - Fatigue
  - Constipation
  - Cold intolerance
  - Depression (slow movement/speech)
  - Weight gain
  - Menorrhagia/oligo- or amenorrhea
  - Myalgias/arthralgias/paresthesias
  - Hoarseness
- Mental status changes in the elderly

Diagnosis/Evaluation

- Hyperthyroidism
  - Physical findings may include goiter, single/diffuse nodule, proptosis, pretibial myxedema, tachycardia, and shortened relaxation phase of deep tendon reflexes
  - Lab findings include increased free T_4, increased free T_3, and decreased TSH
  - 24-hour radioactive iodine uptake scan will reveal diffusely increased uptake in Graves' disease and focal increased uptake in toxic nodules
- Hypothyroidism
  - Physical findings may include dry skin, coarse hair, goiter, and prolonged relaxation of reflexes
  - Lab findings include decreased free T_4, increased TSH, and elevated lipids
  - Antimicrosomal antibodies will be present in cases of Hashimoto's disease

Treatment

- Hyperthyroidism
  - β-blockers are used to relieve symptoms by inhibiting the adrenergic effects of excess thyroid hormone
  - Propylthiouracil (PTU) and methimazole inhibit T_4 synthesis by blocking production of thyroid peroxidase; PTU also blocks peripheral conversion of T_4 to T_3
  - Radioactive iodine may be used to ablate thyroid tissues in patients who have failed antithyroid medications and have contraindications to surgery
  - Subtotal thyroidectomy is indicated for failure of antithyroid medications, obstructing goiters, or patient preference
- Hypothyroidism
  - Thyroid hormone replacement with levothyroxine is generally recommended for all patients with TSH >10 mU/L and presence of goiter or autoantibodies
  - Starting dose and adjustment rates vary with age, weight, concurrent meds, and pretreatment TSH level
  - Treatment is continued indefinitely for chronic disease

Prognosis/Complications

- Hyperthyroidism
  - Thyrotoxic crisis (fever, tachycardia, extreme agitation, delirium) may occur in untreated patients
  - Hypothyroidism may occur following surgery and/or radio-iodine treatments
  - Severe opthalmopathy may occur in Graves' disease
  - Other sequelae include CHF in elderly patients with underlying heart disease, rapid atrial fibrillation, muscle wasting, and osteoporosis
- Hypothyroidism
  - Myxedema coma (lethargy, coma, respiratory depression) is a life-threatening complication if left untreated
  - Other sequelae include treatment-induced CHF in patients with existing heart disease, infertility, and megacolon

57. Thyroid Disease in Pregnancy

Etiology/Pathophysiology

- Normal pregnancy affects thyroid function tests
  - Thyroid-binding globulin (TBG) is increased by estrogen stimulation of TBG production and decreased TBG degradation
  - Elevated TBG leads to an increase in total T_3 and total T_4, while free T_3, free T_4, and thyroid-stimulating hormone (TSH) remain within the normal range
- Hyperthyroidism complicates 1 in 2000 pregnancies
  - The most common cause is Graves' disease, which is associated with thyroid-stimulating antibodies
  - hCG is weak thyroid stimulator; hyperemesis gravidarum may be caused by high serum hCG and is associated with hyperthyroidism (but rarely requires treatment)
- Overt hypothyroidism is rare because it is highly associated with infertility
- Postpartum thyroiditis occurs in 5–10% of women in the U.S.
  - Occurs in up to 25% of women with type 1 diabetes mellitus
  - Thought to be caused by lymphocytic infiltration of the thyroid gland initially (hyperthyroid phase) followed by a hypothyroid phase until the gland recovers

Differential Dx

- Hyperthyroidism
  - Hyperemesis gravidarum
  - Transient subclinical hyperthyroidism
  - Trophoblastic hyperthyroidism
- Hypothyroidism
  - Depression
  - Anemia
- Postpartum thyroiditis
  - Postpartum depression
  - Subacute lymphocytic thyroiditis (postpartum thyroiditis)
  - Chronic lymphocytic thyroiditis (Hashimoto's disease)

Presentation

- Hyperthyroidism
  - Associated with increased rate of spontaneous abortion, premature labor, and low birth weight
  - Tachycardia (greater than the increase seen in normal pregnancy)
  - Thyromegaly
  - Exophthalmos
- Hypothyroidism
  - Associated with high rate of first trimester spontaneous abortion
  - Typical symptoms of hypothyroidism may be present
- Postpartum thyroiditis
  - Thyrotoxic phase (months 1–4): Small goiter, palpitations, fatigue
  - Hypothyroid phase (months 4–8): Goiter, fatigue, depressive symptoms

Diagnosis/Evaluation

- Hyperthyroidism
  - Lab assessment is important, because many nonspecific symptoms are associated with both pregnancy and hyperthyroidism
  - Radionuclide imaging is contraindicated in pregnancy, making it difficult to determine the exact etiology
  - Low serum TSH (<0.01 mU/L)
  - Increased serum free T_4
  - Serum T_3 to T_4 ratio may be used; a high ratio is consistent with Graves' disease or toxic adenoma; a normal ratio is consistent with subacute lymphocytic thyroiditis
- Hypothyroidism presents with low free T_4 and increased TSH
- Postpartum thyroiditis
  - Diagnosed infrequently because of nonspecific symptoms
  - Should have low threshold to perform thyroid function tests
  - Thyrotoxic phase results in increased free T_4 and low TSH
  - Hypothyroid phase results in low free T_4 and increased TSH
  - Associated with antithyroid peroxidase antibodies

Treatment

- Hyperthyroidism: The goal of treatment is to maintain maternal serum free T_4 in the high normal range by using the lowest possible dose of medication
  - Propylthiouracil (PTU) or methimazole (MMI) may be used; both cross the placenta and may cause fetal hypothyroidism and goiter; some prefer PTU because it does not cross the placenta as readily as MMI
  - β-blockers are an option for symptomatic control
  - Thyroidectomy is an option for noncompliant patients or if drug therapy is too toxic
  - Radio-iodine is absolutely *contraindicated* in pregnancy
- Hypothyroidism: The goal of treatment is to normalize maternal serum TSH by daily thyroxine (T_4) supplementation
  - Majority of women require increased T_4 replacement
  - Measure TSH at 4–6 week intervals after medication dose changes and at least once every trimester if stable
- Treat postpartum thyroiditis based on the presenting phase

Prognosis/Complications

- Hyperthyroidism
  - If untreated, there is a high incidence of pre-eclampsia and heart failure
  - Rarely, thyroid storm may occur
  - 1–5% of neonates born to Graves' disease mothers have hyperthyroidism due to transplacental transfer of TSH receptor-stimulating antibodies
- Hypothyroidism
  - If untreated, there is a high incidence of pre-eclampsia, placental abruption, low birth weight, and stillbirth
  - There is some evidence that the mental development of fetus may be affected
- Postpartum thyroiditis
  - Women are at high risk for developing permanent hypothyroidism and should be followed for return to normal function

58. Gallbladder Disease

Etiology/Pathophysiology

- Cholelithiasis (gallstones) and biliary colic (intermittent stone obstruction at the neck of the gallbladder, causing episodic pain)
  - 90% of gallstones are composed of cholesterol; 10% are pigmented stones
  - Risk factors for stone formation include obesity, age >40, female sex, pregnancy (increases with parity), oral contraceptives and hormone replacement, drugs (e.g., fibrates, ceftriaxone, octreotide), total parenteral nutrition, rapid weight loss (e.g., following gastric bypass), cirrhosis, Crohn's disease, and ethnicity (western European, Hispanic, and Native American)
- Acute cholecystitis is infection and inflammation of the gallbladder, thought to occur secondary to partial or complete obstruction of the cystic duct
  - >95% of cases are associated with gallstones
  - Acalculous cholecystitis occurs in severely ill ICU patients; less common in women; not associated with gallstones

Differential Dx

- Choledocholithiasis
- Cholangitis
- Pancreatitis
- Peptic ulcer disease
- Gastritis
- Renal calculi
- Hepatitis
- Right lung pneumonia
- Appendicitis
- Fitz-Hugh-Curtis syndrome
- Intestinal obstruction
- Perforated viscus
- Angina/MI

Presentation

- Most gallstones are asymptomatic
- Biliary colic results in right upper quadrant or epigastric pain
  - May radiate to back or right shoulder
  - Often occurs after a fatty meal
  - Intermittent and resolves spontaneously
  - Crescendos in 15 minutes but may last up to 3 hours
- Acute cholecystitis
  - RUQ pain or epigastric pain as above, but constant and severe
  - Suspect if pain lasts over 4–6 hours
  - Fever, nausea/vomiting, jaundice
  - Gallbladder may be palpable/painful
  - Murphy's sign: Palpation of the right upper quadrant during inspiration results in inspiratory arrest secondary to pain

Diagnosis/Evaluation

- Appropriate history and physical is highly suggestive of gallbladder disease
- CBC will reveal leukocytosis
- Elevations of LFTs, amylase, bilirubin, and alkaline phosphatase may represent choledocholithiasis (stones in the common bile duct)—immediate decompression of the biliary tree is necessary via ERCP, percutaneous transhepatic cholangiogram (PTC), or open common bile duct exploration
- Ultrasound is the gold standard for diagnosis of gallbladder pathology: May show distended gallbladder, thickened walls, pericholecystic fluid, and stones
- Hepatobiliary nuclear scan (HIDA) may be used if the diagnosis is in doubt; examines for cystic duct obstruction and/or acute cholecystitis
- CT may be used but it is somewhat less accurate and much more expensive than ultrasound

Treatment

- Avoid fatty foods and other triggers of biliary colic
- Asymptomatic cholelithiasis need not be treated
  - Consider cholecystectomy in immunocompromised or diabetic patients who have asymptomatic stones due to possible "silent" disease
- Administer IV fluids and broad-spectrum antibiotics (e.g., ampicillin, first-generation cephalosporin, and metronidazole) for patients with cholecystitis
- Cholecystectomy is the treatment of choice for symptomatic cholelithiasis and cholecystitis
  - Laparoscopic (preferable) or open
  - Intra-operative cholangiogram should be used if there is a history of elevated LFTs or amylase, suspicion of choledocholithiasis, or if the ductal anatomy is unclear
  - Lithotripsy may be used to break up stones in patients who are not surgical candidates

Prognosis/Complications

- Very good prognosis if treated early
- Complications include abscess formation, perforation, and formation of a cholecystoenteric fistula with subsequent gallstone ileus
- Complications of cholecystectomy include wound infection, bleeding or hematoma formation, subphrenic or subhepatic abscess, and bile leak (cystic duct leak or injury to common bile duct)
- Though many people have asymptomatic cholelithiasis, few cases will result in cholecystitis—however, once infection occurs, surgery to remove the gallbladder is indicated, as cholecystitis is likely to recur

59. Irritable Bowel Syndrome

Etiology/Pathophysiology

- Etiology is unclear
  - Multicomponent model currently favored
  - Cognitive: Coping strategies
  - Behavioral: Stress from environment (including certain foods)
  - Emotional: Psychological stress, anxiety, depression
  - Physiologic: Neuroendocrine disorder, altered pain modulation, altered motility modulation
- Often presents prior to age 50; 50% present before age 35
- More common in females
- Prevalence thought to be 10–20% in the general population; however, only 30% of patients seek treatment
- Abdominal pain is thought to be secondary to visceral pain hypersensitivity
- Motility problems occur secondary to enhanced gut activity to food and emotional stress
- Dysregulation of the brain-gut axis may play a role as well

Differential Dx

- Secretory diarrhea (e.g., laxative abuse)
- Osmotic diarrhea (e.g., lactose intolerance)
- Inflammatory diarrhea (e.g., ulcerative colitis, Crohn's disease)
- Fatty diarrhea (e.g., short bowel syndrome, pancreatic insufficiency)
- Infectious diarrhea (e.g., *Clostridium difficile* colitis)
- Celiac sprue
- Endometriosis

Presentation

- Abdominal pain predominant variant
- Diarrhea-predominant variant
  - Small- to moderate-volume loose stool
  - Occurs only while awake
  - Associated with meals
- Constipation-predominant variant
- Often aggravated by stress or emotional situations
- Other GI symptoms include nausea, dyspepsia, and dysphagia
- Chest pain may occur
- Pertinent negatives: Patients are *not* awakened at night, not associated with weight loss

Diagnosis/Evaluation

- Rome I criteria (1999): At least 12 weeks of continuous, recurrent abdominal pain that is relieved by defecation, and/or associated with a change in the consistency of stool, and/or associated with a change in the frequency of stool
- Rome II criteria (1999): As above but also requires two or more of the following more than 25% of the time: Altered stool frequency (>3x/day or <3x/week); altered stool form (hard or watery/loose); altered stool passage (incomplete evacuation, straining); mucus; abdominal distension and bloating
- Laboratory studies may include TSH, CBC, electrolytes, glucose, BUN/creatinine, and celiac sprue testing
- Stool studies for stool osmotic gap and weight
- Colonoscopy or sigmoidoscopy in patients >50 (concern for neoplasm) or if concern for inflammatory bowel syndrome

Treatment

- Treat diarrhea symptoms with loperamide (2–4 mg QID as needed), cholestyramine (4 gm Q4h PRN), or alosetron (a $5HT_3$ antagonist only approved in women with diarrhea predominant variant who have failed all other options)
- Treat constipation with fiber, osmotic laxatives, and tegaserod (a $5HT_4$ antagonist approved for short term use only in females)
  - Avoid cathartic laxatives (chronic use worsens problem)
- Treat abdominal pain with antispasmodics (e.g., dicyclomine, hyocyamine) or tricyclic antidepressants (e.g., amytriptiline)
- Use antidepressants for associated depression or anxiety
- Strong doctor-patient relationship is necessary
- Disease has no cure; need to set goals of symptom management
- Coping strategies, behavioral modification
- Dietary modification is helpful: Recommend a low-fat, low-alcohol, low-caffeine diet

Prognosis/Complications

- After 5 years, 5% of patients have complete recovery and 30% of patients have partial recovery

60. Headache

Etiology/Pathophysiology

- Tension headaches are the most common type of headache
  - Originally thought to be caused by muscle tension; however, data now suggests that a vasodilatory component may be responsible
  - Usually present later in the day and relieved with exercise
- Migraine headache is associated with cerebral vasoconstriction followed by vasodilatation
  - May be preceded by an aura (a transient set of neurologic symptoms), most commonly a scotoma (wavy lines across visual field) or focal numbness or weakness
  - May be exacerbated by higher levels of estrogen (e.g., menarche, menstruation, oral contraceptives, pregnancy, hormone replacement therapy); however, menopause, despite decreasing estrogen levels, may also worsen migraines
- Cluster headaches may be associated with decreased regional blood flow to the hypothalamus
  - Often provoked by alcohol

Differential Dx

- Temporomandibular joint (TMJ) pain
- Chronic sinusitis
- Giant cell arteritis (temporal arteritis)
- Meningitis
- Subarachnoid hemorrhage
- Brain tumor
- Carotid artery dissection
- Glaucoma
- Pheochromocytoma
- Optic neuritis
- Hypertension
- Rebound headaches (caffeine, analgesics)

Presentation

- Tension
  - Band-like feeling around head
- Migraine
  - Begins gradually
  - Intensifies within hours
  - Can be unilateral or bilateral
  - Classic migraine has aura
  - Common migraine is without aura
- Cluster
  - Repetitive, occurs in clusters
  - Pain begins suddenly and peaks within minutes
  - Lasts 30 minutes to 3 hours
  - Begins unilaterally around the eye or temple (retro-orbital)
  - Associated with ipsilateral lacrimation, redness of eye, and sweating; may involve Horner syndrome

Diagnosis/Evaluation

- History should include timing, duration, precipitants, prodrome of headaches, family history, and OCP use
- Physical examination should include a focused neurologic examination (e.g., nuchal rigidity, papilledema, level of consciousness, focal weakness)
- Head CT scan is the imaging study of choice if patients present with concerning symptoms or findings (MRI/MRA is better choice for posterior fossa and vascular lesions)
  - "Worst headache of my life" (rule out subarachnoid hemorrhage)
  - Non-acute headache and unexplained neurologic findings
  - Headache with atypical migraine features (e.g., persistent neurologic findings)
  - Significant changes in typical headache presentation
  - Worsening of headache syndrome despite therapy
  - New onset of headaches in a patient >40
  - Headache occurs with exertion

Treatment

- Tension
  - Abortive therapy consists of relaxation, acetaminophen, and NSAIDs
  - Prophylactic therapy may include tricyclic antidepressants, SSRIs, β-blockers, calcium channel blockers, and antiseizure medications (use cautiously)
- Migraine
  - Abortive agents include acetaminophen, aspirin, NSAIDs, ergotamine, and triptans (e.g., sumatriptan)
  - Prophylactic agents include calcium channel blockers, β-blockers, SSRIs, TCAs, estrogens, and NSAIDs
- Cluster
  - 100% oxygen administration is first-line therapy, with or without sumatriptan; other abortive therapies include caffeine, ergotamines, and NSAIDs
  - Prophylactic agents include calcium channel blockers (e.g., verapamil), prednisone, ergotamines, indomethacin, and lithium (use cautiously)

Prognosis/Complications

- Complete recovery should be expected from each episode; however, each of these types of headaches can increase in frequency, duration, and pain
- Should changes in frequency, duration, or pain occur without clear explanation, further evaluation is warranted

61. Back Pain

Etiology/Pathophysiology

- The specific anatomic cause of back pain is often impossible to define, and only a small percentage of patients have an identifiable underlying cause
- A comprehensive history and physical examination can identify the small percentage of patients with serious conditions that require immediate further evaluation
- Back pain occurs at some time during pregnancy in approximately half of women
    - Lumbar lordosis becomes markedly accentuated during pregnancy and may contribute to the development of low back pain
    - In addition, the hormone relaxin softens the ligaments around the pelvic joints and cervix, and this laxity may cause pain by an exaggerated range of motion

Differential Dx

- Back strain
- Acute disc herniation
- Osteo-arthritis
- Spinal stenosis
- Spondylolisthesis
- Ankylosing spondylitis
- Infection
- Malignancy
- Referred pain from other organ systems

Presentation

- Patients should be asked about constitutional symptoms and the presence of night pain, bone pain, or morning stiffness
- Patient should be asked about the occurrence of visceral pain; symptoms such as numbness, weakness, radiating pain, and bowel or bladder dysfunction
- It is also important to inquire about the specific characteristics and severity of the pain, a history of trauma, previous therapy and its efficacy, and the functional impact of the pain on the patient's work and activities of daily living
- "Red flags" include age >50 years, fever, weight loss, bladder/bowel dysfunction

Diagnosis/Evaluation

- Thorough neurologic examination to assess deep tendon reflexes, sensation, and muscles strength
- CBC, ESR, and other specific tests should be ordered as indicated by the clinical evaluation
- Plain-film radiography is rarely useful in the initial evaluation of back pain
- MRI and CT scanning have been found to demonstrate abnormalities in asymptotic patients; thus, positive findings in patients with back pain are frequently of questionable clinical significance; these studies should be considered in patients with worsening neurologic deficits or a suspected systemic cause of back pain such as infection or neoplasm

Treatment

- 2–3 days of bed rest in a supine position is recommended for patients with acute radiculopathy; activity adjustment is preferred for patients with non-neurogenic pain
- Acetaminophen or NSAIDs are the mainstay of pharmacologic therapy; however, NSAIDS are contraindicated in pregnancy
- Superficial heat can be used for analgesia and reduction in muscle spasm; ultrasound can be used for analgesia, by increasing the length of peri-articular ligaments and tendons
- Cold packs can be used for analgesia and limitation of edema in acute musculoskeletal injuries
- Exercise programs that facilitate weight loss, trunk strengthening, and the stretching appear to be most helpful in alleviating low back pain
- Patients with suspected cauda equina lesions, worsening neurologic deficits, or intractable pain should undergo surgical evaluation

Prognosis/Complications

- Approximately 90% of adults in the U.S. experience back pain at some time in life
- This ailment has a benign course in 90% of patients
- As many as 90% of patients with acute back pain return to work within 3 months
- The treatment plan should be reassessed in patients who do not return to normal activity within 4–6 weeks
- Fewer than 2% of patients have disc herniation

62. Depression

Etiology/Pathophysiology

- Many factors in women may contribute to depression, including genetic, biologic, developmental, reproductive, and hormonal (e.g., premenstrual syndrome, childbirth, infertility, menopause) factors
- Women develop their sense of self through nurturing and relationships with others; these traits are devalued in society, which places women at risk of valuing themselves less highly
- Certain personality characteristics (e.g., pessimistic thinking, low self-esteem, sense of having little control over life events, tendency to worry excessively) increase the likelihood of developing depression
- The lifetime prevalence of depression in women is approximately 20% (women experience depression twice as often as men)
- Depression occurs most frequently in women aged 25–44
- Risk factors include family or personal history of mood disorders, history of physical or sexual abuse, loss of social support system, and use of oral contraceptives (especially those with high progesterone content)
- Age of onset may be earlier in women than men and duration of episodes in women tend to be longer with more frequent recurrences
- Depression in women is misdiagnosed in 30–50% of cases

Differential Dx

- Seasonal affective disorder
- Premenstrual dysphoric disorder (PMDD)
- Dysthmic disorder
- Anemia
- Thyroid dysfunction
- Oral contraceptive use
- Medications (e.g., β-blockers, reserpine)
- Drug or alcohol abuse
- Eating disorders
- Somatization disorder
- CNS neoplasms
- SLE
- Lyme disease
- HIV encephalopathy

Presentation

- Depressed mood
- Flat affect
- Poor eye contact
- Appetite or weight changes
- Loss of interest in previously pleasurable activities
- Sleep disturbances (insomnia, hypersomnia)
- Decreased energy or unexplained fatigue
- Decreased libido
- Women are more likely to present with symptoms of atypical depression (e.g., hypersomnia, hyperphagia, weight gain, a heavy feeling in the arms and legs, evening mood exacerbations, insomnia)

Diagnosis/Evaluation

- Guidelines recommend early therapy based on clinical presentation
- Rule out medical illnesses if inadequate response to therapy: CBC, thyroid function tests, vitamin B_{12} level, liver function tests, toxicology screen if appropriate, ANA, HIV if high risk, and Lyme titers
- DSM IV criteria for diagnosis of major depression requires at least five of the following criteria during a 2-week period
  - Depressed mood or inability to experience pleasure
  - Appetite disturbance
  - Sleep disturbance
  - Psychomotor disturbance
  - Fatigue or loss of energy
  - Feelings of worthlessness or excessive guilt
  - Decreased ability to concentrate
  - Recurrent thoughts of death or suicidal ideation
- These symptoms must not be accounted for by bereavement, general medical condition, medications, or drug/alcohol abuse
- Symptoms must result in significant impairment of social, occupational, or school functioning

Treatment

- Depression may respond to individual psychotherapy or cognitive-behavioral therapy, either alone or in combination with pharmacotherapy
- Selective serotonin reuptake inhibitors (SSRIs) are first-line choices (e.g., fluoxetine, sertraline, paroxetine, fluvoxamine, citalopram)
  - Common adverse effects include GI upset, sexual dysfunction, and changes in energy level (e.g., fatigue, restlessness)
- Atypical antidepressants (e.g., venlafaxine, bupropion, nefazodone, mirtazapine) may cause less GI upset and sexual dysfunction than SSRIs
- Medications require 2–6 weeks at therapeutic dose levels to observe a clinical response and should be continued for 6–12 months after resolution of symptoms
- Patients with persistent suicidal ideation require hospitalization

Prognosis/Complications

- With appropriate treatment, 70–80% of individuals can achieve significant reduction in symptoms
- Of patients who are untreated, 40% will continue to meet diagnostic criteria and 20% will have partial remission at 1 year
- 50–80% will experience recurrence
- Depression is associated with occupational dysfunction, including unemployment, absenteeism, and decreased work productivity
- Depression may affect patients' abilities to fulfill parental roles
- Women are twice as likely to attempt suicide than men but men are four times more likely to die from suicide

63. Anxiety Disorders

Etiology/Pathophysiology

- It is hypothesized that pathologic anxiety results from disturbances in the cerebral cortex, specifically the limbic system (i.e., hypothalamus, septum, hippocampus, amygdala, cingulate), other neural bodies, and the connections between these structures
- Major neuroendocrine mediators of anxiety: norepinephrine and serotonin
- Anxiety disorders are the most common mental illness in the U.S., affecting 13.3% of the adult population (ages 18–54)
- Most anxiety disorders begin in childhood, adolescence, or early adulthood
- The female-to-male ratio for any lifetime anxiety disorder is 3:2
- Women and men are equally likely to suffer from obsessive-compulsive disorder and social phobia
- The postpartum period is a time of increased vulnerability to panic disorder and obsessive-compulsive disorder
- DSM IV anxiety disorder include generalized anxiety disorder (GAD), panic disorder with or without agoraphobia, obsessive-compulsive disorder (OCD), post-traumatic stress disorder (PTSD), acute stress disorder, social phobia, and specific phobias (e.g., agoraphobia)

Differential Dx

- Substance-induced anxiety disorder
- Exogenous corticosteroids
- Panic attack
- Hyperthyroidism
- Hypoglycemia
- Ischemia or myocardial infarction
- Arrhythmias
- Pheochromocytoma
- Cushing syndrome
- Withdrawal syndromes

Presentation

- Tremulousness
- Insomnia
- Shaking
- Irritability
- Restlessness
- Muscle tension
- Dry mouth
- Diaphoresis
- Sweaty palms
- Nausea
- Diarrhea
- Urinary frequency
- Excessive worry
- Difficulty concentrating
- Palpitation
- Chest pain
- Numbness (with hyperventilation)

Diagnosis/Evaluation

- History should include a review of medications, caffeine-containing beverages and supplements, and herbal supplements (especially for ephedrine)
- Complete physical exam
- Mental status exam
- Laboratory studies include CBC, chemistries, serum and urine toxicology screens, and thyroid function tests
- Generalized anxiety disorder is defined as persistent fear, worry, or tension in the absence of panic attacks, lasting for at least 6 months
- Obsessive-compulsive disorder is characterized by obsessions or compulsions, which must be recognized as unreasonable or excessive and causes marked distress
- Panic attacks are recurrent episodes of spontaneous, intense periods of anxiety, usually lasting <1 hour and accompanied by at least four of the following symptoms: Palpitations, diaphoresis, tremulousness, shortness of breath, chest pain, dizziness, nausea, abdominal discomfort, fear of injury or going crazy, derealization, and depersonalization

Treatment

- Discontinue (or decrease to a reasonable level) caffeine-containing products (e.g., coffee, tea, cola, chocolate)
- Consider need for psychiatric evaluation
- Cognitive behavioral therapy, interpersonal, or psychodynamic therapy may be helpful
- Benzodiazepines may be used for rapid control of panic attacks, acute situational anxiety disorder, and adjustment disorder in situations when the duration of pharmacotherapy is anticipated to be 6 weeks or less (use with caution due to abuse potential)
- Specific pharmacologic indications include: Generalized anxiety disorder (venlafaxine, buspirone, and paroxetine); social phobia (paroxetine); obsessive-compulsive disorder (fluoxetine, sertraline, paroxetine, and fluvoxamine); and post-traumatic stress disorder (sertraline)
- Inpatient care should be considered if suicide is a risk or detoxification is needed for comorbid substance dependence

Prognosis/Complications

- Untreated panic attacks will usually subside spontaneously within 20–30 minutes, especially with reassurance and a calming environment
- Early treatment improves prognosis and limits social and occupational impairment
- The prognosis for recovery depends on the specific disorder, the severity of symptoms, and the specific causes of the anxiety
- Complications of anxiety disorders include sedative abuse, substance abuse, depression, occupational impairment, and marital and familial difficulties

64. Diabetes Mellitus

Etiology/Pathophysiology

- Type 1 diabetes occurs due to dysfunction of β-cell insulin production
  - Type 1a: Autoimmune destruction of the insulin-producing β-cells in the islets of Langerhans, leading to absolute insulin deficiency; associated with a genetic susceptibility that is triggered by one or more environmental agents (e.g., viral infection, foods, perinatal factors, pre-eclampsia, neonatal respiratory disease, jaundice, high birth weight, long birth length)
  - Type 1b: Idiopathic destruction of the insulin-producing β-cells; no evidence of autoimmunity and no other known cause for β-cell destruction
- Type 2 diabetes is much more common than type 1
  - Characterized by abnormal insulin secretion and peripheral tissue insulin resistance
  - Risk factors include obesity, habitual physical inactivity, family history of diabetes mellitus in a first-degree relative, high-risk ethnic or racial group (e.g., black, Hispanic, Native American), history of high birth weight infant (>9 lb) or gestational diabetes, hypertension, dyslipidemia, impaired glucose tolerance or impaired fasting glucose, and polycystic ovary syndrome

Differential Dx

- Type 1 diabetes
- Type 2 diabetes
- Cushing syndrome
- Acromegaly
- Glucagonoma
- Hyperthyroidism
- First-degree hyperaldosteronism
- Somatostatinoma
- Drugs or chemicals
- Infections
- Genetic defects of β-cell function or insulin action
- Genetic syndromes (e.g., Turner or Down syndromes)

Presentation

- Many women are asymptomatic or present with mild symptoms and are only detected by screening
- Polydipsia or excessive thirst
- Polyuria
- Weight loss
- Visual blurring
- Polyphagia
- Diabetic coma
- Signs of end-organ damage may include micro-albuminuria, nephropathy, proliferative and nonproliferative retinopathy, and retinal hemorrhage

Diagnosis/Evaluation

- Fasting plasma glucose is used to evaluate for diabetes
  - Normal fasting plasma glucose is <110 mg/dL
  - Impaired fasting glucose is 110–125 mg/dL
  - Diabetes mellitus is diagnosed by fasting glucose ≥126 mg/dL or a random blood glucose ≥200 mg/dL
- Initial labs should include CBC, urinalysis, routine blood chemistries (glucose, BUN/creatinine, electrolytes), lipid profile (total cholesterol, HDL, triglycerides), Hb_{A1c}, and an electrocardiogram
- Assess cardiovascular risk: Major risk factors include diabetes mellitus, age >55, dyslipidemia (high LDL and/or low HDL), family history of premature coronary disease (first-degree male relative <55 or female <65), smoking, hypertension, and peripheral vascular disease
- Assess target organ damage: Retinopathy, neuropathy, nephropathy, foot ulcers

Treatment

- Type 1: Patient education on proper diet, exercise, and insulin administration; intensive insulin therapy
- Type 2: Patient education, lifestyle modification (weight loss, exercise, appropriate low sugar diet), oral hypoglycemic agents (sulfonylureas, meglitinides, biguanides, thiazolidinediones, α-glucosidase inhibitors, lipase inhibitors) and exogenous insulin preparations
- Regular screening and risk factor reduction is necessary for all diabetic patients
  - Vigorous cardiac risk reduction (weight loss, exercise, smoking cessation, daily aspirin, angiotensin-converting enzyme inhibitor use to protect kidneys)
  - Routine renal, retinal, and foot examinations
  - Optimal treatment of hypertension and hyperlipidemia
  - Regular blood glucose self-monitoring and improved glycemic control (goal of Hb_{A1c} <7%)
  - Appropriate vaccinations (influenza, pneumococcus)
- Avoid hypoglycemia

Prognosis/Complications

- Acute complications include diabetic ketoacidosis and hyperosmolar coma
- Chronic complications include macrovascular disease, microvascular disease, diabetic foot ulcers, gastroparesis, and sexual dysfunction
  - Macrovascular complications include cardiovascular disease (myocardial infarction, ischemic changes on EKG, heart failure, and peripheral vascular disease)
  - Microvascular complications include retinopathy, nephropathy, and neuropathy
- Appropriate treatment and good glycemic control (Hb_{A1c} <7%) results in decreased incidence and progression of microvascular, but not macrovascular, complications

65. Diabetes in Pregnancy

Etiology/Pathophysiology

- Diabetes mellitus (DM) may exist before pregnancy (types 1 or 2) or develop during pregnancy (gestational diabetes)
- Gestational diabetes mellitus (GDM) refers to carbohydrate intolerance that begins during pregnancy; the prevalence varies in direct proportion to the prevalence of type 2 diabetes in a given population or ethnic group
- The placenta secretes diabetogenic hormones, including growth hormone, corticotropin-releasing hormone, placental lactogen, and progesterone
- If the woman's pancreas is unable to overcome the placenta- and fetal-induced insulin resistance, gestational diabetes develops
- Risk factors for gestational diabetes include family history of diabetes, age >25 years, polycystic ovary syndrome, prepregnancy weight ≥110% of ideal body weight, history of abnormal glucose tolerance, previous unexplained perinatal loss or birth of a malformed child; higher incidence in Hispanic, Native American, or African-American race
- Proposed mechanisms by which hyperglycemia leads to dysmorphogenesis (fetal abnormalities) in the fetus include up-regulation of an apoptosis regulatory gene in the blastocyst stage and creation of excess oxygen radicals that inhibit prostaglandin synthesis

Differential Dx

- Glucose intolerance
- Type 1 diabetes mellitus (juvenile, insulin-dependent)
- Type 2 diabetes mellitus (usually non-insulin-dependent)
- Gestational diabetes mellitus

Presentation

- Approximately 4% of pregnancies are complicated by diabetes
  - 88% of cases are gestational diabetes
  - 4% of cases are type 1 diabetes
  - 8% of cases are type 2 diabetes
- Gestational diabetes is usually an asymptomatic condition and presents at screening at 24–28 weeks gestation
  - 50 gm oral glucose challenge is administered; if serum glucose is ≥140 mg/dL at 1 hour post-challenge, proceed to glucose tolerance test (GTT)
  - Diagnosis requires that two or more thresholds be met or exceeded: 95 mg/dL, fasting; 180 mg/dL at 1 hour; 155 mg/dL at 2 hours; 140 mg/dL at 3 hours

Diagnosis/Evaluation

- Preconception screening of diabetics should include blood pressure, ophthalmologic, cardiac, renal, and thyroid evaluation
- Assess baseline renal function with an early morning urine microalbumin or a 24-hour urine collection for total protein excretion and creatinine clearance
- Laboratory studies include blood glucose measurements 4–8 times daily at home, Hb_{A1c} every 4–6 weeks, urinalysis every 1–2 weeks, check urine ketones to detect ketoacidosis during acute illness or when blood glucose is >200 mg/dL, and serum creatinine each trimester
- Fetal survey ultrasound at 18 weeks to assess for congenital anomalies; repeat ultrasound at 28–30 weeks to assess fetal growth and redo survey
- Twice weekly antepartum fetal testing after 35 weeks; sooner for women with prior DM or poorly controlled GDM who require insulin or have hypertension or adverse obstetric history; GDM is managed the same as women with prior DM; there is no consensus regarding antepartum testing in controlled GDM

Treatment

- Fetal organogenesis is nearly complete at 7 weeks postconception; prepregnancy counseling and glycemic control is essential to reduce congenital malformations
- Diet recommendation is 30 kcal/kg/day for women at ideal body weight
- Goal plasma glucose: Fasting 60–95 mg/dL; 1-hour postprandial <140; 2-hour postprandial <120
- Begin insulin regimen if diet does not control glucose
  - Oral antidiabetic agents are contraindicated in pregnancy as they cross the placenta and may cause fetal hyperinsulinemia and possible teratogenicity
- For nonreassuring antepartum fetal testing, correct reversible causes; if uncorrectable, proceed to delivery; consider delaying delivery long enough to accelerate lung maturity with corticosteroids
- Maternal diabetes alone is not an indication for C-section; C-section may be indicated for macrosomia (fetal weight ≥4,500 gm) to reduce the risk of brachial plexus injury

Prognosis/Complications

- Pre-existing DM: Major congenital malformations occur in 13% of infants born to diabetic mothers (compared with 2% for non-diabetic mothers); neonatal complications include preterm birth, polyhydramnios, macrosomia +/- birth injury, polycythemia, hyperbilirubinemia, cardiomyopathy, metabolic abnormalities, respiratory problems, and growth restriction; maternal complications include pregnancy-induced hypertension, diabetic ketoacidosis, worsening diabetic retinopathy in women with tight glycemic control, and declining renal function
- GDM recurs in 33–50% of subsequent pregnancies; increased risk of hypertensive disorders in pregnancy and DM later in life, neonatal hyperbilirubinemia, macrosomia

66. Hypertension

Etiology/Pathophysiology

- Normal blood pressure: Systolic <120 mmHg and diastolic <80
- Prehypertension BP: Systolic 120–139 or diastolic 80–89
- Stage 1 hypertension: Systolic 140–159 or diastolic 90–99
- Stage 2 hypertension: Systolic ≥160 or diastolic ≥100
- 60% of women >70 years old have hypertension; 50% of women ages 40–70 have hypertension
- 80% of all patients with isolated systolic hypertension are women
- Essential hypertension is associated with increased salt intake, excess alcohol intake, family history of hypertension, obesity, and black race

Differential Dx

- Essential hypertension
- Secondary hypertension
  - Primary renal disease
  - Oral contraceptives
  - Primary hyperaldosteronism
  - Cushing syndrome
  - Pheochromocytoma
  - Hypothyroidism
  - Hyperthyroidism
  - Hyperparathyroidism
  - Sleep apnea
  - Coarctation of the aorta
- Pre-eclampsia

Presentation

- Usually asymptomatic
- Headaches, epistaxis, dizziness, palpitations, and easy fatigability may be present
- Signs of end-organ damage may be present
  - Left ventricular hypertrophy
  - Angina pectoris
  - Congestive heart failure and associated symptoms (e.g., dyspnea)
  - Hematuria
  - Weakness or dizziness due to transient ischemic attacks
  - Chest pain due to coronary artery disease or dissection of the aorta
  - Blurring of vision due to retinopathy

Diagnosis/Evaluation

- Physical exam should assess for end-organ damage (retinopathy, heart failure, left ventricular hypertrophy); auscultate for renal, aortic, or carotid bruit; palpate peripheral pulses, and complete a full neurologic examination
- Initial labs may include urinalysis and routine blood chemistries (creatinine, electrolytes) to assess for nephropathy; blood glucose, lipid profile, and electrocardiogram to assess for cardiovascular risk and left ventricular hypertrophy
- Major risk factors for cardiovascular disease include personal history of coronary heart disease (CHD), age over 55, dyslipidemia: high LDL and/or low HDL, family history of premature CHD (first-degree male relative under age 55 or a female under age 65), diabetes mellitus, smoking, hypertension, peripheral vascular disease

Treatment

- Lifestyle changes may include weight loss; sodium restriction; moderate alcohol consumption; adequate potassium, calcium, and magnesium consumption; smoking cessation; increased physical activity; reduced intake of saturated fat and cholesterol
- Pharmacologic therapies may include thiazide diuretics, β-blocker, ACE inhibitor, angiotensin II receptor blocker, calcium channel blocker, β-1 adrenergic blocker
  - Initial therapy for uncomplicated hypertension is usually a diuretic or β-blocker
  - Patients with diabetic nephropathy: ACE inhibitor
  - Patients with heart failure: ACE inhibitor, diuretics
  - Patients with isolated systolic hypertension: Diuretics or, less preferable, a long-acting dihydropyridine
  - Patients with prior MI: β-blocker without intrinsic sympathomimetic (e.g., metroprolol) activity
  - Patients with left ventricular hypertrophy: Angiotensin II receptor blocker

Prognosis/Complications

- Coronary artery disease
- Stroke or transient ischemic attacks
- Intracerebral hemorrhage
- Left ventricular hypertrophy
- Heart failure
- Ventricular arrhythmias
- Sudden cardiac death
- Benign nephrosclerosis
- Chronic renal insufficiency
- End-stage renal disease
- Peripheral vascular disease
- Retinopathy
- Hypertensive emergencies
- Malignant hypertension
- Goal of drug therapy BP <140/90 (<130/80 with DM or kidney disease)

67. Chronic Hypertension in Pregnancy

Etiology/Pathophysiology

- Chronic hypertension is defined as hypertension (BP >140/90) that is present before pregnancy or that is diagnosed before the 20th week of gestation; hypertension that persists for more than 42 days postpartum is also classified as chronic hypertension
- Chronic hypertension complicates 5–10% of all pregnancies
- Peripheral vascular resistance falls during pregnancy due to the smooth muscle relaxation induced by progesterone, resulting in a progressive fall in blood pressure during the first 24 weeks of pregnancy
- Many women are unaware of hypertension preceding pregnancy, as they have not had regular medical care; since blood pressure naturally falls during the first trimester, hypertension is often not recognized until the second trimester as blood pressure begins to rise
- Risk factors include obesity, African-American race, advanced age, and genetic predisposition

Differential Dx

- Gestational hypertension
- Pre-eclampsia
- Viral hepatitis
- Acute fatty liver of pregnancy
- Gallbladder disease
- Glomerulonephritis
- SLE exacerbation
- Autoimmune thrombocytopenia

Presentation

- Chronic hypertension (diagnosed by BP measurement)
  - Clinical presentation is often missed if the patient presents in the first trimester when blood pressure normally falls
  - Chronic hypertension is present if blood pressure is high in the first trimester
  - Symptoms may include headache, dizziness, visual changes, abdominal pain, and lower extremity edema
- Gestational hypertension is associated with the above symptoms during the third trimester

Diagnosis/Evaluation

- Chronic hypertension
  - Elevated blood pressure during the first 20 weeks of gestation or preceding the pregnancy
  - Normal renal studies
  - Normal liver function tests
  - Normal blood count
- Gestational hypertension
  - Elevated blood pressure after the first 20 weeks of gestation
  - No symptoms of pre-eclampsia

Treatment

- Chronic hypertension may be treated with labetalol, hydralazine, nifedipine, methydopa, or β-blockers
  - Diuretics may be continued if already used prior to the pregnancy; however, they should not be initiated during pregnancy
  - ACE inhibitors are contraindicated in pregnancy; associated with fetal and neonatal renal failure and death
- The above treatments are also appropriate for gestational hypertension

Prognosis/Complications

- 85% of patients with chronic hypertension have normal pregnancies; the majority of pregnant women with chronic hypertension have uncomplicated mild hypertension and can be managed the same as normal, non-hypertensive women during the intrapartum period
- Associated with a higher incidence of perinatal death (4.5%), small for gestational age infants (16%), cesarean section (30%), and pre-eclampsia (5–18% incidence, which results in the poorest fetal outcomes)
- Antihypertensive therapy does not prevent pre-eclampsia

68. Obesity

Etiology/Pathophysiology

- Obesity is a complex, multifactorial condition in which excess body fat may put a person at health risk
- Obesity is defined as a BMI >30.0
- BMI is defined as a person's weight in kilograms divided by the square of the person's height in meters
- Excess body fat results from an imbalance of energy intake and physical expenditure
- Energy needs vary by age and gender and are also affected by body size and composition, genetic factors, co-existing pathologic conditions, ambient temperatures, and physiologic states such as growth, pregnancy, and lactation
- Waist circumference measurements >102 cm in men or 89 cm in women indicate an increased risk of obesity-related co-morbidities
- Recommended weight gain during pregnancy is determined by prepregnant BMI. It is recommended that overweight women gain 6.8–11.4 kg (15–25 lbs) while obese women should gain 6.8 kg (15 lbs)

Differential Dx

- Underweight = BMI <18.5
- Normal = BMI 18.5–24.9
- Overweight = BMI 25.0–29.9
- Obesity class I = BMI 30.0–34.9
- Obesity class II = BMI 35.0–39.9
- Obesity class III = BMI >40

Presentation

- Patients may present with obesity-related complications, including osteo-arthritis, gallstones, sleep apnea, and infertility
- Physicians should assess their patients for overweight and obesity during routine medical examinations and discuss with at-risk patients the health consequences of further weight gain

Diagnosis/Evaluation

- Assessment requires determination of the degree to which a person is overweight and a patient's overall risk status
- This determination encompasses evaluation of total body fat, abdominal body fat, and various risk factors for diseases and conditions associated with obesity including a family history of obesity-related disease
- BMI is significantly correlated with total body fat content and should be used to assess overweight and obesity as well as to monitor changes in body weight
- Abdominal fat content should be assessed before and during weight loss treatment by measurement of waist circumference

Treatment

- Treatment is recommended for patients with a BMI of 25.0–29.9 kg/m^2 or a high waist circumference and two or more risk factors; treatment is also recommended for patients with a BMI >30 kg/m^2 regardless of risk factors
- Overweight persons without risk factors should be encouraged to avoid further weight gain
- Treatment goals are to reduce body weight, maintain a lower body weight over the long term, prevent further weight gain, and control accompanying disease risk factors
- Effective medical approaches include dietary therapy, increasing physical activity, behavior therapy, pharmacotherapy, and combinations of these techniques
- Weight loss drugs should only be used as part of a comprehensive treatment program; currently, FDA-approved drugs include sibutramine (an appetite suppressant) and orlistat (a lipase inhibitor)

Prognosis/Complications

- Heart disease
- Type 2 diabetes mellitus
- Hypertension
- Stroke
- Certain types of cancer (endometrial, breast, colon)
- Dyslipidemia
- Gallbladder disease
- Sleep apnea and other respiratory problems
- Reduced fertility
- Osteo-arthritis
- Increase in all cause mortality
- Emotional distress
- Discrimination
- Social stigmatization

69. Epilepsy

Etiology/Pathophysiology

- Epilepsy is a syndrome of recurrent seizures
- 3% cumulative incidence of seizures by age 80
- Prevalence of 5–8/1000 people (0.5–0.8%)
- Peak ages of onset are in girls <10 and women >60
- Etiologies include idiopathic (e.g., juvenile myoclonic epilepsy), cryptogenic (unknown), symptomatic (e.g., secondary to a brain lesion or systemic disease), and congenital (e.g., cortical dysplasia, heterotopia)
- Catamenial epilepsy is seizure activity related to the menstrual cycle
  - High estrogen-progesterone ratio during menstrual cycle causes frequent seizures (estrogen is proconvulsant; progesterone is an anticonvulsant)
  - 75% of women with epilepsy have exacerbations related to menstrual cycle
- Women with epilepsy have higher rates of infertility, sexual dysfunction, ovarian cysts, osteoporosis, and menstrual irregularities; in addition, some anti-epileptic drugs affect oral contraceptive pill efficacy
- 50% of women with epilepsy have increased seizure frequency during pregnancy (due to changes in pharmacokinetics, sleep deprivation, nausea)
- Menopause may worsen or improve epilepsy; combination HRT is helpful

Differential Dx

- Syncope (pale skin, arrhythmias, and postural symptoms are more associated with syncope than seizures)
- Vasovagal episode
- Hypoglycemia
- Pseudoseizures
- Anxiety attack

Presentation

- Partial seizures (with focal onset)
  - Partial simple: Focal symptoms
  - Partial complex: Focal symptoms with altered alertness
- Generalized seizures (generalized onset with loss of consciousness)
  - Grand mal: Convulsive
  - Tonic: Spasm of face and trunk with flexion of upper limbs and extension of lower limbs
  - Clonic: Rhythmic movements
  - Myoclonic: Quick muscle jerks
  - Atonic: Sudden loss of muscle tone
  - Bilateral movements are always associated with loss of consciousness (LOC)
  - Petit mal: Nonconvulsive
  - Absence seizure: Eyes blinking, staring

Diagnosis/Evaluation

- Obtain a complete history of the event, including information from witnesses if possible
  - Note presence of aura (aura is a visual, auditory, or other focal symptom perceived at seizure onset)
  - Tongue or cheek biting, urinary incontinence, confusion after the event, and headache are more common in seizure and uncommon in syncope
  - Note history of head trauma, cancer, stroke, and infection
  - Note family history of siblings with seizures or neurologic diseases
- Physical examination should include pattern of injury, inspection of skin, and complete neurologic exam (focal deficit may suggest brain lesion or postictal "Todd's Paralysis" phenomena)
- Laboratory evaluation may include EEG, MRI with contrast (provides better resolution than CT to identify smaller brain abnormalities), toxicology screen, and anti-epileptic drug levels

Treatment

- Folate supplementation for women of childbearing age
- Closely monitor anti-epileptic drug serum levels
- Vitamin K replacement during third trimester
  - Anticonvulsant therapy in pregnancy has been associated with hemorrhagic disease (deficiency in neonatal coagulation factors II, VII, IX, and X, with normal levels of factors V, VIII, and fibrinogen), which is a pattern that is similar to vitamin K deficiency
  - Evidence suggests vitamin K supplements prevent this complication
  - Pregnant women with epilepsy should receive oral vitamin K beginning at 36 weeks gestation
  - Newborns should receive intramuscular vitamin K immediately after delivery
- Changes in medical therapies may increase seizure frequency and should be avoided after the first trimester; goal is monotherapy using the lowest efficacious dose

Prognosis/Complications

- 90% of epileptic women have healthy pregnancy outcomes
- Fetal malformations (congenital heart disease, neural tube defects, cleft palate and lip) occur at double the rate of the general population (4–6%), regardless of antiseizure medication use
- Preconception folic acid supplementation (4 mg) is recommended to prevent neural tube defects, which occur more frequently in offspring of epileptic women
- Fetal hydantoin syndrome (growth and mental deficiencies, microcephaly, dysmorphic facial features) occurs in 11% of fetuses exposed to anti-epilepsy drugs
- Risk of congenital malformation is 4–8% with use of first-generation anticonvulsants (2–4% risk in the general population)

70. Deep Venous Thrombosis

Etiology/Pathophysiology

- Deep venous thrombosis (DVT) is defined as one or more blood clots in deep vein(s) of the extremities or the pelvis
- The most life-threatening complication is a pulmonary embolism
- Proximal DVTs are more likely to embolize
- Risk factors include immobility, trauma with injury to vessel walls (especially long bone fractures), previous DVT, pregnancy, estrogen use, age >40 years, indwelling catheters, cancer, hypercoagulability, and polycythemia
- Oral contraceptives increase the risk of DVT, especially in women who smoke
- Hormone replacement therapy increases the risk of DVT and is not recommended in women with previous DVT or hypercoagulability
- Factor V Leiden is the most common hereditary blood coagulation disorder in the U.S.; it is present in 5% of the Caucasian population and 1.2% of the African-American population
- Most often, DVT is associated with a hypercoagulable state in addition to a risk factor

Differential Dx

- Cellulitis
- Lymphedema
- Compression of a vein by a mass or enlarged nodes
- Muscle injury
- Superficial thrombophlebitis

Presentation

- Many cases are asymptomatic
- Limb pain and/or swelling
- Homan's sign: Pain upon dorsiflexion of foot
- Palpable cord in affected extremity
- Redness of extremity
- Fever
- Pulmonary embolism may present with tachycardia, shortness of breath, and sharp chest pain

Diagnosis/Evaluation

- Doppler ultrasound is the most widely used diagnostic technique; it is noninvasive and highly sensitive and specific for popliteal and femoral thrombi
- Venography is the most sensitive and specific test but is technically difficult and uncomfortable for the patient
- Impedance plethysmography has equal sensitivity and specificity to Doppler ultrasound
- Laboratory studies may be indicated to evaluate for a hypercoagulable state: Factor V Leiden and antithrombin III are the most common; protein C and S and antiphospholipid antibodies are less common
- D-dimer test is positive in the face of any clotting; a negative D-dimer is helpful to rule out DVT, but a positive test does not rule it in

Treatment

- Prophylaxis against DVT is indicated in patients having major surgery, myocardial infarction, stroke, and in patients who are immobile for prolonged periods
- Above the knee thromboses are treated with IV heparin (initial bolus of 80 U/kg followed by 15–18 U/kg/hr); then administer warfarin 5–10 mg/day 1–3 days after heparin therapy is initiated (note that warfarin is teratogenic); bed rest is indicated to prevent embolism
- Below the knee thromboses: Treated as an outpatient with leg elevation and NSAIDs, or Lovenox SQ 2x/day (dosed by weight) and Warfarin (does not require apt testing, also used for above the knee), or as an inpatient with IV heparin
- Inferior vena cava filter may be indicated in patients with a contraindication to anticoagulation or repeated thrombosis despite adequate anticoagulation
- Consider long-term low-dose warfarin to prevent recurrence

Prognosis/Complications

- 20–25% of untreated proximal DVTs result in pulmonary embolism
- Pulmonary embolism has a 15–20% mortality rate
- Anticoagulation therapy decreases the risk of pulmonary embolism 10-fold
- Post-phlebitic syndrome: Pain and edema in the extremity with no evidence of continuing clot
- Complications of anticoagulation therapy include hemorrhage and stroke
- Women who are heterozygous for factor V Leiden have a 20–30-fold increased risk of thrombosis if they take combined oral contraceptives; the risk does not appear to be elevated with progestin-only contraceptives

71. Thrombosis in Pregnancy

Etiology/Pathophysiology

- Numerous changes in the coagulation system and physiologic changes in the body account for the hypercoagulable state associated with pregnancy: Increased venous stasis, increased capacity and distensability of veins, increase in clotting factors (I, VII, IX, X), decrease in fibrinolytic activity, resistance to activated protein C, decrease in protein S, and increased activation of platelets
- Up to half of women who have thrombotic events in pregnancy possess an underlying thrombophilia; the most common thrombophilias include factor V Leiden mutation and prothrombin gene mutation F20210A
- Risk factors include prolonged bed rest, cesarean section, multiple pregnancies, obesity, and advanced maternal age
- Antepartum deep vein thrombosis is as common as postpartum thrombosis and occurs with equal frequency in all three trimesters; pulmonary embolism is more common in the postpartum period
- Other sites of thrombosis in pregnancy include the pelvic veins, subdural clots, and cavernous sinus thrombosis

Differential Dx

- Edema of pregnancy
- Superficial thrombosis
- Chronic venous stasis changes

Presentation

- Lower extremity venous thrombosis: Unilateral pain, edema, redness, and warmth in lower extremity
- Pulmonary embolism: Acute shortness of breath, tachycardia, anxiety, and hypoxia

Diagnosis/Evaluation

- Duplex Doppler ultrasonography
- Compression ultrasound: Uses firm compression with the ultrasound transducer probe to detect an intraluminal filling defect
- Impedance plethysmography: Measures impedance flow with pneumatic cuff inflation around the thigh
- Venography: If clinical suspicion is high and noninvasive test results are negative, limited venography with abdominal shielding is indicated
- For the diagnosis of pelvic vein thrombosis and internal iliac thrombosis, MRI may be used, but its role is still not well defined in pregnant women
- Pulmonary embolism has traditionally been evaluated with ventilation-perfusion scanning (V/Q); this results in minimal radiation exposure to the fetus (<0.1 rads); however, approximately 40–60% are nondiagnostic in pregnancy
- Spiral CT may be useful for diagnosing pulmonary embolism

Treatment

- Antepartum thrombosis
  - Anticoagulation with unfractionated IV heparin initially, then subcutaneous heparin
  - Low molecular weight heparin may be an alternative
  - Coumadin is embryotoxic and therefore contraindicated in pregnancy
- Postpartum thrombosis
  - IV unfractionated heparin initially, then coumadin for 3 months
  - Coumadin does not interfere with breast-feeding
  - Inferior vena cava filter insertion may be used if anticoagulation is contraindicated (e.g., inherited bleeding disorders, active GI bleeding, hemorrhagic stroke, recurrent emboli despite anticoagulation)

Prognosis/Complications

- Pulmonary embolism
- Increased risk of recurrence
- Post-thrombotic syndrome (subcutaneous tissue with edema, ulceration or impaired viability)
- Treatment complications include osteopenia (due to heparin) and bleeding

72. Mitral Valve Prolapse

Etiology/Pathophysiology

- The mitral valve consists of the leaflets, the annulus, the chordae tendinae, and papillary muscles, as well as the supporting left ventricular wall
- Mitral valve prolapse (MVP) is a billowing of one or more of the mitral valve leaflets into the left atrium during systole; may occur with or without mitral regurgitation
- Primary MVP occurs with myxomatous proliferation of the spongiosa of the valve; etiologies include idiopathic, genetic, and connective tissue diseases (e.g., Marfan syndrome)
- Secondary MVP is not a primary valve leaflet problem (i.e., not associated with myxomatous degeneration); common causes include coronary artery disease and coronary ischemia, and papillary muscle rupture, resulting in a flail mitral leaflet, rheumatic heart disease, hypertrophic cardiomyopathy, and annulus dilatation
- Affects 15 million people in the U.S. (2–6% of women and men alike); the most common congenital heart lesion found in women of childbearing age
- May result in mitral regurgitation (MR)

Differential Dx

- Mitral regurgitation
- Other valve abnormalities (e.g., aortic or pulmonic clicks)
- Cardiac ischemia

Presentation

- Asymptomatic in many patients
- Palpitations (often without evidence of arrhythmias or tachycardia)
- Chest pain
- Anxiety
- Panic attacks
- Exercise intolerance
- Orthostatic hypotension
- MVP syndrome: Patients have the above symptoms but it is unclear what the physical etiology is, or whether it is truly associated with MVP
- Severe (usually late stage disease) MVP is associated with arrhythmias (e.g., atrial fibrillation) and shortness of breath (due to CHF or pulmonary hypertension)

Diagnosis/Evaluation

- Physical examination reveals a midsystolic click, best heard at the apex (may be intermittent), and a late systolic murmur
  - Look for pectus excavatum, scoliosis, and arachnodactly, which suggest a connective tissue disease as the etiology
  - Squatting results in an increase in left ventricular volume, which causes the click to occur later in systole (closer to S2)
  - Standing, isometric hand grip, and Valsalva maneuver results in a decrease in left ventricular volume, causing the click to occur earlier (closer to S1)
  - Significant MR may result in orthostatic hypotension
- EKG is most often normal, but can rarely show T wave abnormalities or ST depressions; QT prolongation is also seen
- Echocardiogram is not necessary if only a click is heard on exam; if a murmur is present, echo will assess the excursion of the valve leaflets, LA and LV sizes, and LV function
  - Serial echos are not necessary for asymptomatic patients
- Cardiac catheterization is only indicated in patients with severe MR, symptomatic MR, or decreased LV dysfunction, prior to possible valve repair or replacement

Treatment

- Asymptomatic MVP requires only reassurance and follow up every 2–3 years
- Endocarditis prophylaxis (amoxicillin 2 gm PO 1 hour prior to procedure) is indicated only if a murmur indicates MR or if there is valve thickening (not needed if only a click is present); there is a debate whether to prophylax women undergoing vaginal or cesarean delivery
- Symptomatic patients with palpitations, chest pain, or anxiety should avoid caffeine, alcohol, and tobacco; may respond to β-blockers; liberal fluid and salt intake with compression stockings; administer mineralocorticoids if required; aspirin should be given to those patients with neurologic events, but is not recommended in others
- Surgery is reserved for patients with severe MR, LV dysfunction, atrial fibrillation, and/or elevated pulmonary pressures; mitral valve repair tends to be very successful; most patients do not require replacement

Prognosis/Complications

- Complication rate of <2% per year
- Complications are related to severity of MR
  - Arrhythmias: Ventricular ectopy and sudden death; atrial fibrillation due to left atrial dilatation
  - Left ventricular dysfunction and CHF
  - Pulmonary hypertension
  - Right ventricular dysfunction
  - Infective endocarditis
- Neurologic events (TIA) may be linked, though this is questionable
- MVP is the most common cause of MR in pregnancy
  - Pregnancy can improve symptoms with increased blood volume and decreased peripheral vascular resistance (PVR)
  - Pregnancy is well tolerated in most women; there is concern only if there is a decreased LV ejection fraction

73. Tobacco Abuse

Etiology/Pathophysiology

- The most common tobacco used by women is cigarettes
  - Cigar, pipe, and smokeless tobacco use among women is low
  - Cigar use has risen to 9.8% in adolescent girls
- Smoking initiation is usually due to social and familial factors, while nicotine dependence is what keeps people smoking
- Smoking is the major preventable risk factor for coronary heart disease
- 25% of American women of reproductive age smoke
- Smoking remains the leading cause of death and preventable death in women
- Lung cancer is the leading cause of cancer deaths in women, largely attributed to cigarette use
- Smoking is an important modifiable risk factor associated with adverse pregnancy outcomes
  - About 12–22% of pregnant women smoke cigarettes
- Pathophysiology of tobacco-induced adverse fetal outcomes
  - Nicotine-induced vasospasm decreases placental perfusion
  - Carboxyhemoglobin diminishes oxygen delivery to the fetus
  - Direct toxicity of nicotine, ammonia, vinyl chloride, and any of the other 2500 substances found in cigarettes

Differential Dx

- DSM IV nicotine-related disorders
  - Nicotine use disorder
  - Nicotine dependence
  - Nicotine-induced disorder
  - Nicotine withdrawal
- Marijuana abuse
- Alcohol abuse
- Illicit drug abuse
- "Casual cigarette use"

Presentation

- Routine health maintenance exam
- Acute illness visit
- Tobacco-induced health problem
- Prepregnancy planning
- Infertility visit
- Prenatal visit
- Specifically for tobacco cessation therapy

Diagnosis/Evaluation

- Screen patient for readiness to quit at each visit
- Stages of change model applies to smoking cessation
  - Precontemplation
  - Contemplation
  - Preparation
  - Action
  - Maintenance
  - Relapse
- Counsel pregnant smokers at first prenatal visit and throughout the course of pregnancy
  - Quitting early in pregnancy provides the most benefit to the fetus and mother
  - Quitting late in pregnancy can still provide some benefit

Treatment

- About 3/4 of smoking women say they want to quit smoking, and about half have tried in the previous year
- Cessation programs yield a 20–40% 1 year abstinence rate
- Therapies include self-help, psychological therapy, group programs, nicotine replacement systems (patch, gum, nasal spray), and pharmacotherapy (bupropion)
- Set specific quit date, +/- pharmacologic agents
- Counsel on weight gain; methods to reduce weight gain (exercise, low cal snacks, planned activities for hands to avoid eating)
- Nicotine replacement systems (gum, spray, patch) for women with nicotine addiction (usually smoking 1.5 packs/day); start with higher dose on quit date, taper slowly over 3–6 months
- Sustained-release bupropion effective for all levels of smoking and may prevent weight gain
- Pharmacotherapy should be considered in pregnancy if unable to quit

Prognosis/Complications

- Women smokers who die of a smoking-related disease lose 14 years of potential life
- Women who stop smoking reduce their risk of dying prematurely; benefits of smoking cessation are greater when women stop at younger ages, but it's beneficial at all ages
- COPD, pneumonia, and influenza
- Lung cancer; cervical cancer; oral cavity, larynx, esophagus, bladder, kidney, pancreas, and stomach cancers
- Coronary artery disease
- In pregnancy related to intrauterine growth restriction; spontaneous abortion; placenta previa; placental abruption; premature rupture of the membranes; low birth weight
- Eliminating maternal smoking: 10% reduction in infant deaths; 12% reduction in infant deaths from perinatal conditions

74. Alcohol Abuse

Etiology/Pathophysiology

- A maladaptive pattern of alcohol use leading to clinically significant distress in a 12-month period (DSM IV criteria)
- About 10% of women will meet the criteria for alcohol abuse in their life
- 13.5% of women binge drink (defined as five or more drinks on one occasion within the past 30 days)
- 3–5% of women have alcohol dependence
- A childhood history of attention deficit/hyperactivity disorder or a current diagnosis of a personality disorder (antisocial personality disorder) predisposes to alcohol-related disorders
- There is a significant genetic component: 3–4-fold increased risk of an alcohol-related disorder if there is a first-degree relative with an alcohol-related disorder; higher concordance rate among separated monozygotic twins
- 1 out of every 50 pregnant women consume at least five or more drinks at least once during their pregnancy
- Fetal alcohol syndrome is defined as brain disorders, growth retardation, and facial malformations resulting from inutero exposure to alcohol

Differential Dx

- Alcohol intoxication
- Alcohol dependence
  - Early stage problem drinkers (do not yet have complete dependence)
  - Affiliative drinkers (drinks daily in moderate amounts in a social setting)
  - Schizoid isolated drinkers (severe dependence, drinks alone, and binge drinks)

Presentation

- Acute intoxication
- Acute withdrawal
- Inpatient and postoperative withdrawal symptoms in unsuspecting patients
- Routine health maintenance screening
- Prenatal screening
- Medical complications

Diagnosis/Evaluation

- Use the four-step "Ask, Assess, Advise, and Monitor" model for screening and brief intervention
- **CAGE** scale is used to assess drinking behavior
  - Have you ever felt you ought to **Cut** down on your drinking?
  - Have people **Annoyed** you by criticizing your drinking?
  - Have you ever felt **Guilty** about your drinking?
  - Have you ever had a drink upon waking in the morning to steady your nerves or get rid of a hangover (an "**Eye-opener**")?
  - 1 point for each affirmative answer; positive test if the patient scores ≥2 points
- Screen for complications of alcohol abuse based on extent of abuse and presenting symptoms
  - Liver disease (fatty liver, hepatitis, cirrhosis)
  - Gastrointestinal disorders (gastritis, esophagitis, pancreatitis)
  - Nutritional deficiencies (vitamin B_{12} or folate deficiency)
  - Neuropathy
  - Cardiovascular disease (hypertension, cardiomyopathy)

Treatment

- Inpatient pharmacologic management of acute alcohol withdrawal
  - Treat tremulousness and agitation with chlordiazepoxide (Librium) or diazepam (Valium)
  - Treat hallucinations with lorazepam (Ativan)
  - Treat withdrawal seizures with diazepam
  - Treat delirium tremens with lorazepam
- Pharmacologic management for abstinence
  - Disulfiram (Antabuse) inhibits acetaldehyde dehydrogenase; 10–15 mL of ingested alcohol will produce an uncomfortable reaction (headache, sweating, vomiting, tachycardia, and vertigo)
  - Naltrexone (opiate-receptor antagonist) reduces relapse in alcohol-dependent adults
- Complete abstinence from alcohol is the goal of treatment
- Alcoholics Anonymous meetings may be useful

Prognosis/Complications

- The life expectancy of alcoholic women is reduced by more than 15 years
- Causes of death linked to alcohol abuse include cirrhosis, pancreatitis, cancer, cardiovascular disease, unintentional injury, suicide, and violence
- Drunk driving is associated with half of all automotive fatalities
- Fetal alcohol syndrome and alcohol-related neurodevelopmental disorders occur in 9.1 per 1,000 live births
- Fetal alcohol syndrome is the leading cause of mental retardation in the U.S.

75. Substance Abuse

Etiology/Pathophysiology

- The DSM IV definition of substance abuse is a maladaptive pattern of substance use, leading to clinically significant impairment or distress, as manifested by one or more of the following, occurring in a 12-month period:
  - Recurrent substance use resulting in a failure to fulfill major role obligations at work, school, or home
  - Recurrent substance use in situations in which it is physically hazardous
  - Recurrent substance-related legal problems
  - Continued substance use despite having persistent or recurrent social or interpersonal problems caused or exacerbated by the effects of the substance
  - The symptoms above never met the criteria for substance dependence
- Substance dependence is more severe and may include tolerance and withdrawal
- Alcohol, amphetamines, cannabis, cocaine, hallucinogens, inhalants, opioids, phencyclidine, and sedatives are substances of abuse
- The rate of illicit drug use in American women is about 4.5%
- Women abuse prescribed drugs more often then men (Vicodin, Fiorinal)
- Illegal substance exposure in childbearing women is approximately 11%

Differential Dx

- Substance use
- Substance dependence
  - Behavioral
  - Physical
- Substance intoxication
- Substance withdrawal
- Depression
- Anxiety

Presentation

- Polysubstance abuse: ≥12 months of repeated substances used from at least 3 categories (not nicotine or caffeine)
- Acute intoxication; acute withdrawal
- Injury, medical complications (hepatitis, chest pain), concerns addressed by family members
- Depression and weight control problems may present as over-the-counter stimulant, cocaine, or amphetamine abuse
- Routine health maintenance exam; specifically as a reason for therapy; failed drug test screen
- Suspect substance abuse in pregnancy: Late presentation for prenatal care; multiple missed prenatal visits; previous unexplained miscarriage, prematurity, or congenital anomalies

Diagnosis/Evaluation

- Diagnosis can be made by screening for substance abuse during routine health maintenance exams and prenatal visits
- The major goal of the initial evaluation is for the patient to trust the physician and end up committed to an appropriate and workable treatment
- Stages of change model to assess patient's readiness to quit
  - Precontemplation
  - Contemplation
  - Preparation
  - Action
  - Maintenance
  - Relapse
- Urine drug screens

Treatment

- Goals of treatment: Abstinence; physical, psychiatric, and psychosocial well being
- Inpatient therapy is indicated for
  - Severe medical symptoms associated with withdrawal
  - Severe psychiatric symptoms associated with withdrawal
  - History of failed outpatient therapy
  - Lack of psychosocial supports
  - Severe or long-term history of substance abuse
- After initial detoxification, patients require sustained rehabilitation
  - Individual, family, and group therapy
  - Education about substance abuse
- In some cases pharmacotherapy may be needed to control withdrawal symptoms or to sustain abstinence: Alcohol: disulfiram (inhibits acetaldehyde dehydrogenase); opiates: methadone (to reduce the effect of withdrawal and cravings); reassess patient's commitment to abstinence throughout and after therapy
- Reassess patient's commitment to abstinence throughout and after therapy

Prognosis/Complications

- Only 20–50% of patients remain abstinent during the first year after treatment
- Social complications include:

  - Divorce   – Debt
  - Incarceration   – Violence

- Medical sequelae depend on the type of abused drug, but include
  - Psychiatric disorders
  - Cardiovascular disease (including hypertension, myocardial infarction)
  - Infectious disease
  - Sexual dysfunction
  - Death
- Perinatal complications of drug use include

  - Low birth weight   – Preterm delivery
  - Placental abruption   – Congenital anomalies
  - Mental retardation   – Miscarriage
  - Sudden infant death syndrome

76. Sexual Assault

Etiology/Pathophysiology

- Sexual assault is defined as any sexual act performed by one person on another without consent; rape and sodomy are components of sexual assault
- Rape is defined as the perpetration of an act of sexual intercourse with a person against her will and consent
- The perpetrator of rape may overcome the victim by force, by fear from the threat of force, or with drugs/intoxicants
- Statutory rape is defined as vaginal penetration of a child who is younger than 18 years old
- Date rape is a term applied to rape in which the rapist is known to the victim
- Wife rape (spousal rape) occurs when a woman is sexually assaulted by her husband or ex-husband without consent or against her will
- Sodomy is defined as forced acts of fellatio or anal penetration
- 1 in 3 women will be a victim of sexual assault
- 1 in 4 women will experience rape or attempted rape during college
- 50–80% of rape victims know their assailant
- Sexual assault accounts for 7% of all violent crimes in the U.S.
- Among battered women, approximately 35% experience marital rape

Differential Dx

- Physical abuse
- Emotional abuse
- Sexual abuse
- Incest
- Severe emotional distress from accidental or intentional injury

Presentation

- Only half of sexual assault survivors will ever seek help
- <20% of sexual assault victims report to an emergency department for immediate medical attention
- Only 10–15% of sexual assaults are reported to police
- Presenting symptoms range widely from severe emotional disturbance to seeming control and total denial; regardless of presentation, all women should be closely followed for sequelae
- Screening for past sexual assault in primary care may identify victims with chronic emotional sequelae

Diagnosis/Evaluation

- Acute evaluation should be done by specifically trained providers; many institutions have SANE (Sexual Assault Nurse Evaluation) models or similar programs, with providers that are skilled in the collection of forensic evidence and who are sensitive to psychological trauma experienced by victims
- History should focus on explicit details of the assault for forensic purposes and to guide the physical exam
- It is also important to know the activities of the victim after the assault; activities such as bathing, changing clothes, eating, urinating, and using enemas may lower the yield of forensic specimen collection
- A full physical exam, including a description of the patient's emotional state and photographic documentation of any traumatic injuries, is important; the breasts, external genitalia, vagina, and rectum should be carefully examined
- The victim should be counseled about post-coital contraception, STDs (including HIV) and pregnancy testing; screening for date rape drugs should be done if the victim reports amnesia regarding the event

Treatment

- Assess and treat any life-threatening injuries
- Empiric antibiotic therapy may be indicated
  - Gonorrhea: 125 mg single dose IM ceftriaxone
  - Chlamydia: 1gm single dose of oral azithromycin or 100 mg BID of oral doxycycline for 7 days
  - Trichomoniasis: 2 gm single dose of oral metronidazole
- Administer hepatitis B vaccination with or without hepatitis B immunoglobin in victims who have not already been vaccinated against hepatitis B
- Prophylactic treatment of HIV should be offered
  - 300 mg of zidovudine and 150 mg of lamivudine BID for 4 weeks works best started within 4 hours of assault
  - Do not prescribe if >72 hours has passed
- Post-coital emergency contraception should be offered
  - 100 μg of ethinyl estradiol plus 0.5 mg of levonorgestrel (or 0.75 mg of levonorgestrel alone)
  - Give at presentation and 12 hours later
  - Best results if used within 72 hours of intercourse

Prognosis/Complications

- 3–16% risk of chlamydial infection, 11% risk of PID, and 7% risk of trichomoniasis
- 0.2% risk of HIV (increased with genital trauma, bleeding, or ulcerative lesions)
- Rape-trauma syndrome may occur
  - The early phase lasts days to weeks; symptoms include anger, fear, anxiety, physical pain, sleep disturbances, anorexia, and intrusive thoughts
  - The late phase is a reorganization phase that can last for months; symptoms include genital, musculoskeletal, and pelvic/abdominal pain
  - Anorexia and insomnia may persist
- Victims may find it difficult to resume their habits, lifestyles, and sexual relationships
- Post-traumatic stress syndrome, depression, or anxiety syndromes may develop

77. Domestic Violence

Etiology/Pathophysiology

- CDC definition of domestic or partner violence: Actual or threatened physical or sexual violence, or psychological/emotional abuse, by a spouse, ex-spouse, boyfriend/girlfriend, ex-boyfriend/ex-girlfriend, or date
- Lifetime prevalence among U.S. women ranges from 25–54%, with 1.5–15% of women reporting having been victimized within the past year
- Partner violence affects all racial and socioeconomic backgrounds, as well as same-sex relationships
- Partner violence occurs commonly during pregnancy (4–8% of pregnancies)

Differential Dx

- Accidental injury
- Depression
- Anxiety
- Munchausen syndrome

Presentation

- Patients who present with injuries should be asked about partner violence, especially if the injuries are suspicious
- Although many victims are injured as a result of partner violence, many will not present for acute medical care; therefore health-care providers should screen all patients for partner violence during routine visits

Diagnosis/Evaluation

- Routine screening for domestic violence in all patients is much more effective than only inquiring when there is suspicion
- The Partner Violence Screen, a short screening tool, is positive for current physical abuse with a "yes" response to any of the following questions:
  - Have you been hit, kicked, punched or otherwise hurt by someone in the past year? If so, by whom?
  - Do you feel safe in your current relationship?
  - Is there a partner from a previous relationship who is making you feel unsafe now?

Treatment

- Acknowledge and validate abuse history
- Perform a safety assessment by evaluating for
  - Imminent threat of violence: Situations associated with heightened danger include change in status of the relationship, substance abuse in the perpetrator, recent escalating violence, history of threats with weapons/possession of firearms, pattern of intense jealousy in the perpetrator
  - Suicidality
  - Psychological sequelae (e.g., anxiety, depression, post-traumatic stress disorder)
- Provide appropriate referrals and follow up
  - Mental health and domestic violence services
  - Shelters and safe homes
  - Legal advocacy services
  - Hotlines (National Domestic Violence Hotline: 1-800-799-SAFE)

Prognosis/Complications

- Survivors of partner violence are more likely to have more general health problems resulting in worse health status and greater disability, more mental health problems resulting in higher levels of depression and anxiety, and increased healthcare utilization and higher annual healthcare costs

Pregnancy

MARY BETH GORDON, MD
MELODY YEN HOU, MD
NGOC T. PHAN
HOPE A. RICCIOTTI, MD

Section 6

78. Maternal Physiology

Cardiovascular
- Normal physiologic changes of pregnancy include reduced exercise tolerance, jugular venous distension, peripheral edema, systolic ejection murmur (96%), and S_3 gallop (90%)
- Central hemodynamic changes: Blood volume is increased by 40%; cardiac output is increased 40% by 24 weeks; heart rate is increased by 15%
- Blood pressure is decreased due to the vasorelaxant effect of progesterone until 24 weeks; systemic vascular resistance is decreased by 21%; pulmonary vascular resistance is decreased by 35%; systolic blood pressure is decreased by 5–10 mmHg; diastolic blood pressure is decreased by 10–15 mmHg
- EKG reveals left axis deviation

Respiratory
- 65% of women perceive dyspnea
- Nasal edema, congestion, epistaxis
- Mechanical changes include rising of the diaphragm by 4 cm, flaring of ribs outward, and increased chest circumference by 5–7 cm
- Pulmonary function changes

Total lung capacity	Increased by 5%	FEV_1	unchanged
Tidal volume	Increased by 40%	Respiratory rate	unchanged
Residual volume	Increased by 20%	Peak flow	unchanged
Minute ventilation	Increased by 40%	Vital capacity	unchanged

- Arterial blood gas

	pH	PaO_2	$PaCO_2$
Nonpregnant	7.40	93–100	35–40
Pregnant	7.40	100–105	28–30

Gastrointestinal
- Nausea ("morning sickness") affects up to 70% of women; peaks at 8–10 weeks; likely due to elevated β-hCG
- Gingivitis
- Peptic ulcer disease: ↓ risk; ↑ gastric mucin; ↓ gastric acid secretion
- Gastroesophageal reflux disease (GERD): ↑ risk; ↓ esophageal motility; ↓ tone of gastroesophageal sphincter
- Constipation (30%): ↓ intestinal motility; hemorrhoids due to ↑ central venous pressure
- Gallstones: ↑ risk due to ↓ emptying of gallbladder; ↑ biliary cholesterol saturation
- Liver: Size unchanged; ↑ alkaline phosphatase due to production by placenta; ↓ albumin by 25% due to hemodilution

Renal
- Kidneys increase in size by 1 cm; pelvicalyceal dilation occurs by 15 mm on right, 5 mm on left; ureteral diameter increases by 2 cm (right > left, likely due to mechanical compression by the enlarging uterus)
- Pyelonephritis: Increased risk
- Filtration: Renal flow is increased by 75% by 16 weeks; glomerular filtration rate increases by 50% by 12 weeks; creatinine clearance increases by 40%; glucose excretion increases (1–10 gm/day); protein loss is unchanged

Hematology
- Increased plasma volume by 30–34 weeks of 50%
- Increased erythrocyte mass by 18–30%
- Because of this hemodilution, the hematocrit drops during a normal pregnancy; at 12 weeks, the mean hemoglobin is 12.2 gm/dL; at 28 weeks, the mean is 11.8 gm/dL; at 40 weeks, the mean is 12.9 gm/dL
- Peripheral white blood cell count rises progressively during pregnancy: first trimester range is 3,000–15,000/mm³; in the second and third trimesters the range is 6,000–16,000/mm³; in labor the count may rise to 20,000–30,000/mm³
- There is a progressive decline in platelet count throughout pregnancy, although in the healthy gravida the count will remain within the normal range for nonpregnant subjects
- Pregnancy has been called a hypercoagulable state; increased levels of fibrinogen (factor I) and factors VII–X rise progressively throughout pregnancy

Endocrinology
- The maternal thyroid gland is increased in size but the normal pregnant woman is euthyroid; there is estrogen-induced synthesis of thyroxine-binding globulin, resulting in increases in total T_3 and T_4; free T_4 remains unchanged; maternal TSH, T_3, and T_4 do not cross the placenta, but the thyroid-stimulating immunoglobulins cross readily
- Adrenal glands: Cortisol production is increased and DHEAS is decreased
- Pregnancy is a diabetogenic state: Increased insulin resistance (50–80% decreased insulin sensitivity), decreased peripheral glucose uptake, decreased fasting glucose; increased lipolysis due to human placental lactogen

79. Fetal Physiology

Cardiovascular
- Fetal circulation establishes at approximately 6 weeks gestation to bring oxygen and nutrients from the mother via placental transfer and to discharge waste
- The umbilical vein carries oxygenated blood from the placenta to the fetus. It travels through the liver as the ductus venosus and connects directly to the IVC, transporting oxygenated blood to the right atrium
- The portal vein connects to the umbilical vein
- The fetal lungs are filled with water and do not provide any oxygenation. Blood that enters the right atrium via the IVC is diverted to the left atrium through a patent foramen ovale. The remaining blood exits the right ventricle, into the pulmonary arteries. Most of this blood shunts to the aorta through the ductus arteriosus. The remaining pulmonary artery blood flows to the lungs, and will return deoxygenated to the left atrium
- The systemic circuit includes two umbilical arteries that branch off of the internal iliac. Systemic blood returns deoxygenated to the right heart, where it combines with the oxygenated blood from the umbilical vein
- The fetal heart rate is variable from beat to beat, due to opposing autonomic inputs. This variability can be noted by external fetal heart monitoring and is increased by fetal movement and decreased by acidemia

Respiratory
- Fetal gas exchange occurs in the placenta, with diffusion of carbon dioxide occurring along a concentration and pressure gradient from the fetus to the mother. This is facilitated by the higher oxygen affinity of fetal hemoglobin and higher overall hemoglobin content
- The neuromuscular control of breathing develops in utero, with the movements helping to develop the muscles and respiratory epithelium so they are ready for immediate postnatal use
- Type 2 alveolar cells begin producing surfactant at around 20 weeks, though not in ample quantity for extra-uterine breathing until 28–34 weeks. Surfactant reduces the pressure required to open alveoli during aeration
- Within seconds of delivery, sudden pressure and temperature changes combined with rising carbon dioxide and falling oxygen levels stimulate the first breath. Rising oxygen is thought to activate chemoreceptors in the central respiratory center and local musculature to initiate regular breathing. Amniotic fluid from the lung is absorbed

Gastrointestinal
- The fetal liver is an important hematopoietic organ and stores glycogen and iron. Gluconeogenesis, glucuronidation, and the synthetic functions are not fully developed prenatally. The latter is due in part to vitamin K deficiency (vitamin K is normally produced by intestinal bacteria that are absent in the fetus). These deficiencies predispose the newborn to hypoglycemia, jaundice, and hemorrhage
- Meconium is solid waste that accumulates in the GI tract late in gestation. It is released into the amniotic fluid due to vagally-mediated peristalsis in times of fetal distress or as the normal result of GI maturation at term

Renal
- The fetal kidney does not have responsibility for fluid and electrolyte balance until after birth; it does produce urine as early as 9–12 weeks gestation
- The fetal kidney has immature proximal and distal tubule function, impairing its ability to regulate sodium and acid
- Fetal urine is a primary contributor to amniotic fluid volume (renal agenesis or dysfunction is a primary cause of oligohydramnios)

Central Nervous System
- The central nervous system develops throughout gestation, neonatal, and even adult life
- Maturation can be monitored in part by following fetal movements; they are jerky and basic between 10–20 weeks gestation; from midterm onward, they become more coordinated and patterned
- The fetus acquires swallowing at 10 weeks, breathing movements by 14–16 weeks, primitive sucking by 24 weeks
- Ears and eyes have rudimentary function by 26 and 28 weeks, respectively

Hematology
- Red blood cells (RBCs) are formed first in blood islands in the yolk sac. By 12 weeks gestation, the liver produces most RBCs. The spleen and bone marrow gradually adopt this function, such that at term 90% of RBCs are formed in the marrow
- Hemoglobin F, comprised of two α- and two β-globin chains, is the predominant fetal hemoglobin. It has a higher oxygen affinity than adult (maternal) hemoglobin A and is present in greater concentrations. These factors favor placental oxygen transfer from mother to fetus
- Leukocytes appear in fetal circulation at 8 weeks gestational age. Although developing fetal plasma cells within the spleen and lymph nodes can produce small quantities of IgM and even IgG, production of IgA and IgD does not begin until the first postnatal weeks. The predominant antibody in the fetus is maternal IgG, which crosses the placenta beginning at 16 weeks

Endocrinology
- Fetal endocrine glands develop and actively produce hormones by the end of the first trimester
- Insulin produced by the fetus is a major fetal growth factor; insulin does not cross the placenta
- Evidence suggests steroids produced in the fetal adrenal cortex may initiate labor

80. Prenatal Care

Etiology/Pathophysiology

- Prenatal care is designed for patient education and to screen for complications of pregnancy; important issues include initial evaluation and risk assessment, nutritional counseling, screening for disease (e.g., hypertension, diabetes), and preparing for delivery
- Gravidity refers to the number of times a woman has been pregnant
- Parity refers to the number of pregnancies that led to a birth beyond 20 weeks or of an infant weighing >500 gm
- Abortion is fetal death (therapeutic or spontaneous) before 24 weeks gestation
- Nagele's rule for calculating the estimated date of delivery (EDD): Subtract three months from the last menstrual period (LMP) and add 7 days; exact dating is calculated by 280 days after the last menstrual period
- Pregnancy testing is accomplished by urine test for the β subunit of human chorionic gonadotropin (β-hCG); becomes positive around the time of the missed menses; serum β-hCG becomes positive 1 week after conception
- Ultrasound may be used to determine the EDD: Ultrasound in the first trimester has an error margin of 3–7 days; second trimester has an error margin of 7–10 days; third trimester may be off by as many as 3 weeks

Differential Dx

- Low-risk pregnancy requires only routine prenatal care
- High-risk pregnancy may require maternal fetal medicine co-management or transfer

Presentation

- Prenatal visit schedule: Outpatient appointments every 4 weeks until the 28th week; every 2–3 weeks thereafter until the 36th week; then weekly until delivery
- Uterine size on pelvic exam is accurate for first trimester sizing to confirm gestational age
- Doppler auscultation of fetal heart tones is audible at 10–14 weeks
- Fetoscope heart tones become audible at 19–20 weeks
- Uterus reaches umbilicus at 20 weeks
- Fundal height (pubic symphysis to top of fundus) is an accurate measure of gestational age from 16–38 weeks (fundal height in cm = weeks gestation)

Diagnosis/Evaluation

- History: Last menstrual period, obstetric history (SAB, TAB), and prior deliveries (gestational age, mode of delivery, time in labor, birth weight, complications)
- Physical examination includes complete physical and clinical pelvimetry to assess adequacy of the pelvis for delivery
- Routine prenatal visits include blood pressure, maternal weight, fundal height, fetal heart tones, fetal position, observation for edema, and urinalysis (protein, glucose, blood, and leukocyte esterase)
- Ultrasound will visualize a gestational sac at approximately 5 weeks or at β-hCG of 1,500 mIU/mL; the fetal heart beat may be visible by 6 weeks or β-hCG of 5,000-6,000
- Laboratory studies include CBC, blood type/screen, RPR, rubella antibody, hepatitis B surface antigen, gonorrhea and chlamydia, PPD, Pap smear, urinalysis/culture, varicella titer (if no history of exposure), HIV screening, triple screen (15–18 weeks), fetal survey (18–20 weeks), glucose tolerance test (24–28 weeks), group B streptococcus screen (35–37 weeks)

Treatment

- Improve nutritional and hygienic measures
- The only restrictions in employment are to avoid prolonged standing and strenuous physical work
- During travel, prolonged sitting should be avoided due to risk of thromboembolism (pregnancy is a hypercoagulable state); limit driving to <6 hrs/day; patients should walk for 10 minutes for every 2 hours of driving/sitting; seatbelt should be worn under the abdomen
- There are no restrictions on sexual activity for low-risk patients; however, coitus should be avoided if the patient is at risk for preterm labor
- Review drug and medication usage; only prescribed medications should be taken; avoid teratogens
- Appropriate weight gain during pregnancy is 25–35 lb
- Prenatal exercise should be encouraged
- Breast-feeding should be encouraged
- Encourage childbirth education classes

Prognosis/Complications

- Full term: ≥37 weeks
- Preterm birth: <37 weeks
- Low birth weight: <2500 gm
- Maternal death: Death while pregnant or within 42 days postdelivery/termination
  - Direct: Due to pregnancy state, labor, puerperium
  - Indirect: Due to a pre-existing condition or a condition exacerbated by pregnancy (e.g., pulmonary embolus, hypertension, hemorrhage, infection/sepsis)
- Maternal mortality is reported as number of maternal deaths per 100,000 live births
- Neonatal mortality is reported as neonatal deaths (death <28 days) per 1000 live births
- Perinatal mortality is reported as (fetal deaths plus neonatal deaths) per (1000 live births plus fetal deaths)

81. Prenatal Diagnosis

Etiology/Pathophysiology

- Prenatal diagnosis and genetic counseling is offered to all women who have an increased risk of fetal aneuploidy or anatomic abnormalities: Age >35, abnormal triple screen, more than two miscarriages, previous stillbirth, previous child with birth defects, parental chromosomal abnormality or carrier of genetic disease, and abnormal fetal ultrasound
- Major congenital defects constitute 2–3% of live births; minor defects constitute 5% of live births
  - Causes are chromosomal (0.5%), single-gene defects (1%), and unknown (>60%)
  - Chromosomal abnormalities (e.g., Down syndrome, other autosomal trisomies) increase with maternal age: Age 30 risk is 1/385; age 35 risk is 1/200; age 40 risk is 1/65; age 45 risk is 1/20; 97% occur in families with no previous history of the syndrome
- Triple screen test identifies 60% of Down syndrome and trisomy 18; triple screen plus level II ultrasound detects 85% of Down syndrome; low alpha fetoprotein (AFP) detects 80% of neural tube defects
- A normal fetal anatomy scan in the second trimester reduces the risk of Down syndrome by 45–80%

Differential Dx

- Fetal aneuploidy (chromosomally abnormal fetuses)
- Anatomic abnormalities with normal chromosomes (neural tube defects, cleft lip/palate without associated chromosomal abnormalities)
- Abnormal fetal ultrasound findings but normal chromosomes and normal anatomy (choroid plexus cysts, nuchal lucencies)

Presentation

- Trisomy 21 (Down): Thickened nuchal fold, duodenal/esophageal atresia, atrial/ventricular septal defects; short femur
- Trisomy 18 (Edward): Growth restriction, hydramnios, micrognathia, omphalocele, clubbed feet, diaphragmatic hernia, clenched hands, choroid plexus cysts
- Trisomy 13 (Patau): Cleft lip/palate, holoprosencephalopathy, ventricular septal defect, polycystic kidneys, polydactyly, omphalocele

Diagnosis/Evaluation

- Triple screen is a screening test for neural tube defects (NTD) and chromosomal abnormalities
  - May be done at 15–20 weeks (age must be accurate)
  - Components include AFP, hCG, and estriol; adjusted for maternal age
  - AFP is a fetal glycoprotein related to albumin and produced by the yolk sac, gastrointestinal tract, and liver; if elevated, need to confirm gestational date via ultrasound
  - Elevated AFP is associated with gastrointestinal and genitourinary obstruction, renal disease, skin defects, and hygroma
  - AFP is decreased in trisomies, intrauterine fetal death, obesity, and diabetes
- Diagnostic tests include amniocentesis (performed at 16–18 weeks; 1/250 loss rate) and chorionic villus sampling (performed at 10–12 weeks; 1/100 loss rate)
- Other testing methods include percutaneous umbilical blood sampling, pre-implantation genetic diagnosis, and analysis of fetal RBCs in maternal blood

Treatment

- Prenatal diagnosis is performed for several reasons
  - Helps in making decisions about pregnancy termination
  - May provide useful information for the physician and the patients for planning and management of abnormal neonates
  - If the fetus is found to have aneuploidy or structural abnormalities, management of pregnancy, labor, and mode of delivery can be optimized
  - Some structural defects (such as diaphragmatic hernia) are amenable to experimental fetal surgical interventions

Prognosis/Complications

- If alpha fetoprotein is elevated, gestational age should first be confirmed via ultrasound; inaccurate dates and twins may account for abnormalities
- Amniocentesis results in 0.4% pregnancy loss rate
- Chorionic villus sampling results in 1% pregnancy loss rate

82. Multiple Gestation

Etiology/Pathophysiology

- Twins occur at a spontaneous rate of 1/80 pregnancies; triplets occur in 1/7000 pregnancies; twins are either monozygotic or dizygotic
- Monozygotic twins result when a single fertilized ovum splits into two distinct individuals after a variable number of divisions; dizygotic twins result when two separate ova are fertilized
- Twin placentation: Twin placentas are described in terms of their membranes
  - With a singleton, there is an outer chorion and an inner amnion
  - With dizygous twins, the placentas are always diamniotic-dichorionic
  - With monozygous twins, depending upon the timing of the cleavage of the fertilized ovum, the following possibilities can occur: diamniotic-dichorionic (division occurs during the first 2–3 days); diamniotic-monochorionic (division occurs between 3–8 days); monochorionic-monoamniotic (division occurs between 8–13 days); and conjoined twins (division occurs between 13 and 15 days); beyond 15 days, the process of twinning cannot occur
- The tendency for monozygotic twins does not seem to be heritable; dizygotic twins tend to run in families; other risk factors include advanced maternal age, African descent, and assisted reproduction

Differential Dx

- On ultrasound, retro-membranous collections of blood or fluid or a pronounced fetal yolk sac may make a singleton pregnancy look more like a multiple
- A multiple gestation may be missed due to the second fetal head being tucked in the pelvis or the second heart being obscured

Presentation

- Uterine size greater than dates
- Excessive maternal weight gain
- Palpation of three or more fetal parts or abdominal measurement >4 cm larger than expected value
- Auscultation of more than one fetal heart
- Incidental finding on routine ultrasound
- Elevated maternal serum triple screen values
- Suspicion should be high in any woman who became pregnant with the use of in vitro fertilization or ovulation stimulation

Diagnosis/Evaluation

- On ultrasound, separate gestational sacs can be seen by 6 weeks after the last menstrual period; separate beating fetal hearts can be visualized by 6 weeks on transvaginal ultrasound (8 weeks on abdominal ultrasound)
- Very rarely (with routine prenatal ultrasounds being so common) does diagnosis not take place until the delivery room when another fetal presenting part is palpated after the delivery of the first baby
- Normal individual twins grow at the same rate as singletons up to 30–32 weeks gestation; regular ultrasonic scanning permits ongoing assessment of individual growth; women with multiples should be scanned every 3–4 weeks after the 26th week and more frequently than that if IUGR or growth discordance is suspected

Treatment

- If both twins are vertex (40%), a trial of labor (TOL) is warranted; cesarean section should be performed for the usual obstetrical indications
- If twin A is vertex, but twin B is non-vertex (40%), a TOL can also be attempted providing that the fetuses are 2000–3000 gm and if twin B is equal in size or smaller than twin A; after delivery of twin A, external version can be attempted or vaginal breech extraction can be used to deliver twin B; if twin B is larger than twin A, cesarean delivery may be considered
- The remaining 20% of twins are pregnancies in which twin A is non-vertex and twin B is either vertex or non-vertex; these are delivered by cesarean section
- Triplets are generally delivered by cesarean section; a trial of labor is controversial and is usually only attempted when the fetuses are all concordant and all greater than 1500–2000 gm
- Higher multiple pregnancies always have C-section

Prognosis/Complications

- Increased risk of prematurity; average fetal age at delivery is 36–37 weeks for twins and 33–34 weeks for triplets
- Increased risk for previa, cord prolapse, postpartum hemorrhage, cervical incompetence, gestational diabetes, pre-eclampsia, congenital abnormalities, growth restriction, and malpresentation
- The incidence of growth restriction and fetal death are higher for monochorionic than dichorionic twins; monochorionic twins are at a risk for twin-twin transfusion syndrome, in which arteries in one placenta communicate with veins from the other placenta, manifested by discordance in fetal growth; monoamniotic twins have very high mortality rate (40–60% for one twin) due to cord entanglement

Maternal Complications of Pregnancy

ALISON V. CAPE, MD
MELODY YEN HOU, MD
NGOC T. PHAN
HOPE A. RICCIOTTI, MD

Section 7

83. Bleeding in Early Pregnancy

Etiology/Pathophysiology

- Bleeding in early pregnancy occurs in 20–25% of pregnancies; approximately half of cases ultimately result in a spontaneous abortion
- Implantation bleeding: Caused by invasion of the conceptus into the vascular endometrium; bleeding is minimal and occurs about 2 weeks after conception
- Spontaneous abortion (miscarriage): A pregnancy that ends before 20 weeks gestation; 15–25% of all pregnancies end in miscarriage; 60–80% of cases are associated with abnormal chromosomes
- Missed abortion: Death of the fetus before 20 weeks, with retention of the products of conception in utero
- Incomplete abortion: Occurs when a part of the products of conception have been expelled but some still remain within the uterus
- Ectopic pregnancy: A pregnancy that is implanted outside of the endometrial cavity; approximately 1% of all pregnancies are ectopic, but this figure varies from group to group
- Molar pregnancy: A type of gestational trophoblastic disease in which there is abnormal proliferation of trophoblastic (placental) tissue

Differential Dx

- Threatened abortion
- Implantation bleeding
- Spontaneous abortion
- Incomplete abortion
- Ectopic pregnancy
- Molar pregnancy
- Polyps or fibroids
- Vaginal or cervical lesions/lacerations

Presentation

- Patients present with vaginal bleeding that is observed to be from the cervix
- Bleeding is often light and painless in cases of implantation bleeding and threatened abortions
- Heavy bleeding, passage of tissue, and cramping are usually associated with incomplete and complete abortions
- Ectopic pregnancies usually present with light bleeding accompanied by pain; if the ectopic pregnancy is ruptured, intra-peritoneal hemorrhage may occur, resulting in signs and symptoms of hypovolemia (e.g., hypotension, pallor, weakness) and peritonitis (e.g., rebound tenderness)
- Molar pregnancies usually present with heavy, painless vaginal bleeding

Diagnosis/Evaluation

- Initial evaluation includes a pelvic examination and confirmation of pregnancy with a pregnancy test
- ABO blood typing and screen for irregular antibodies to assess Rh status and to prepare for possible blood transfusion
- CBC is indicated to assess blood loss if bleeding is profuse
- Spontaneous abortion is evaluated by ultrasound; a normal ultrasound that shows the presence of a fetal heart beat decreases the risk of spontaneous abortion to <5%
- Threatened abortion is diagnosed when bleeding is observed to be coming from a closed cervix; it becomes inevitable when the cervix dilates and products of conception are seen passing through the internal os or when the bleeding is profuse
- Complete abortion is noted when the uterus has expelled its contents, the internal os is closed, the bleeding is minimal, and the uterus has returned to near normal size
- Molar pregnancy is classically associated with vaginal bleeding, uterus enlarged beyond the size expected for gestational age, β-hCG levels >100,000 mIU/mL, and ultrasound showing a "snowstorm" appearance

Treatment

- All Rh-negative patients should receive RhoGAM
- Any tissue the patient has expelled should be sent to pathology to assess that products of conception have passed
- Patients with threatened abortion should be observed for continued bleeding; although bed rest is often advised, there is no evidence that this affects the outcome
- Missed abortions often proceed to complete abortions within 1–3 weeks; patients may also be treated by dilatation & evacuation or medical induction of miscarriage with misoprostol
- Incomplete abortions can be allowed to finish or can be completed by dilatation & evacuation
- Ectopic pregnancies are treated surgically or with methotrexate
- Molar pregnancies require dilatation & evacuation with follow-up β-hCG levels for 6 months

Prognosis/Complications

- Approximately half of women who bleed during early pregnancy will go on to have a spontaneous abortion
- Pregnancies that continue have a higher incidence of preterm labor and preterm rupture of membranes
- Spontaneous abortion that is not recurrent (two or more consecutive miscarriages) is not associated with an increased risk of future miscarriage
- Ectopic pregnancies have a recurrence risk of approximately 12–15%
- Recurrence risk of the development of gestational trophoblastic disease in future pregnancies is <5%

84. Bleeding in Late Pregnancy

Etiology/Pathophysiology

- Bleeding after 24 weeks gestation complicates about 5% of pregnancies
- Placental abruption (premature separation of placenta): Constitutes 30% of antepartum bleeding (complicates 1% of all pregnancies); risk factors include previous placental abruption, pre-eclampsia or hypertension, multiparity, trauma, rapid decompression of overdistended uterus (multiple gestations, polyhydramnios), substance abuse (tobacco, alcohol, amphetamines, cocaine)
- Placenta previa (implantation of placenta near or at the cervical os): 20% of antepartum bleeding (present in 0.5% of pregnancies); bleeding is thought to occur in association with the development of the lower uterine segment in the third trimester; placental attachment is disrupted as this area thins in preparation for labor; when found incidentally on ultrasound, 90% of cases will resolve due to placental migration; risk factors include advanced maternal age, multiparity, multiple gestations, and previous C-section
- Vasa previa (fetal vessel rupture over the cervical os): Risk factors include velamentous cord insertion and succenturiate lobes (those separate from the main placenta often connect by fetal vessels protected only by membranes)
- Structural causes of bleeding include cervical polyps, cervical erosion, fibroids, or trauma

Differential Dx

- Placental abruption
- Placenta previa
- Marginal separation
- Gestational trophoblastic disease
- Genital tract lesions
- Bloody show
- Ruptured vasa previa
- Ruptured uterus
- Cervical carcinoma
- Trauma
- Infection

Presentation

- Placental abruption: Painful vaginal bleeding (revealed abruption); bleeding is absent in 20% of cases (concealed abruption); abdominal pain; uterine contractions (hypertonus); tenderness; fetal distress
- Placenta previa: Painless, bright red bleeding (maternal blood); 20% have contractions; usually no fetal distress; fetal malpresentation is common; often detected on ultrasound in the absence of bleeding
  –Total/complete: Placenta covers os
  –Partial: Placenta partially covers os
  –Marginal: Extends to margin of os
  –Low-lying: Within 2–3 cm of internal os
- Vasa previa: Acute vaginal bleeding with associated fetal distress

Diagnosis/Evaluation

- Cervical cultures to rule out infection
- Assess fetal status by non-stress test and biophysical profile
- Amniocentesis for lung maturity if delivery is considered
- Others tests include CBC (to assess anemia), coagulation studies (to assess for DIC), and Betke-Kleihauer test (assess for fetal RBC in maternal circulation if abruption is suspected)
- Placental abruption: Exam reveals contractions (hypertonus), bleeding, abdominal pain, and tenderness; ultrasound may show retroplacental clot with large abruptions, but a normal ultrasound does not rule out the diagnosis
- Placenta previa: Ultrasound is diagnostic (90% of those found in the second trimester will resolve by term due to placental migration); ultrasound should be used assess for placenta previa prior to vaginal or speculum exam
- Vasa previa: Ultrasound is used to diagnose a succenturiate placental cotyledon (one separate from the main placenta) or an anomaly of the umbilical cord insertion; Doppler exam of the membranes over the cervix; Apt, Ogita, or Loendersloot test to distinguish maternal versus fetal blood

Treatment

- Urgent restoration of normal blood volume and coagulation factors is a primary goal in treating obstetrical hemorrhage and DIC
  –Assess volume status by urine output (>30 mL/hr)
  –Replace blood products
- Placental abruption
  –If patient is stable with preterm fetus, no intervention
  –Tocolytics may be used (magnesium sulfate is first choice, has fewer adverse side effects than β-agonists)
  –Frequent fetal monitoring
  –Deliver fetus if moderate to severe abruption (vaginal delivery if fetus stable; cesarean if fetal distress or maternal condition not stable)
  –Give Rh-immune globulin to all Rh-negative patients
- Placenta previa: Bed rest, tocolytics (magnesium sulfate is first choice), and betamethasone; deliver by cesarean section when fetal lung maturity is present
- Vasa previa: Emergent delivery by cesarean section

Prognosis/Complications

- Abruption: Risk of recurrence 5–17%
  –Complications of placental abruption include fetal distress, fetal death, and preterm delivery; maternal complications include hemorrhagic shock, coagulopathy, and renal failure
- Risk of placenta previa in patients with a previous C-section is 1–4%
  –Complications include fetal distress, fetal death, preterm birth, and maternal hemorrhagic shock (DIC is rare)
  –Placenta previa with invasion of uterine wall (10%) is called placenta accreta; associated with prior cesarean section and uterine surgery
- Vasa previa: High fetal mortality (>50%)

85. Ectopic Pregnancy

Etiology/Pathophysiology

- The incidence of ectopic pregnancy is 1–2%, which has increased over the last 10 years due to increased diagnosis and an increase in risk factors
- Responsible for 10% of maternal mortality (mainly due to hemorrhage)
- *Chlamydia trachomatis* infection is the most important risk factor
    - Other risk factors include prior ectopic pregnancy, prior tubal surgery (including sterilization), tobacco use, DES exposure in utero, assisted reproductive technologies, history of sexually transmitted disease or pelvic inflammatory disease, prior abdominal/pelvic surgery (due to adhesions), and endometriosis
    - Douching and early age of first intercourse also slightly increase the risk, but this may be due to associated lifestyles
- More than 95% of ectopic pregnancies are located in the fallopian tube, usually the distal fallopian tube (ampullary portion)
    - Other sites include ovary, cervix, external surface of fallopian tube, abdominal wall, and bowel
- On rare occasions, both intrauterine and extra-uterine gestations can co-exist (heterotopic pregnancy); the risk for this is higher with assisted reproductive technologies, such as in vitro fertilization

Differential Dx

- Intrauterine pregnancy or heterotopic pregnancy
- Incomplete or threatened abortion
- Appendicitis
- Pelvic inflammatory disease/salpingitis
- Ovarian cystic rupture
- Ovarian or tubal torsion
- Kidney stone
- Diverticulitis
- Dysmenorrhea
- Dysfunctional uterine bleeding
- Mittelschmerz

Presentation

- Classic triad of missed menstrual period, irregular vaginal bleeding, and lower abdominal pain
- The most common symptom is sudden, severe, unilateral abdominal pain
    - Pain may radiate to the shoulder
- The most common sign is abdominal tenderness
- Ruptured ectopic pregnancies may present with syncope, shock, and/or peritoneal irritation (e.g., rebound tenderness)

Diagnosis/Evaluation

- History and physical exam is often suggestive of the diagnosis, especially when risk factors are present and the patient presents with a missed period and irregular vaginal bleeding
- Exam may reveal an adnexal mass (possibly tender), a uterus that is small for gestational age, cervical bleeding, decreased blood pressure, and/or shock
- All female patients of childbearing age who present with abdominal pain require immediate β-hCG testing
    - In stable patients without definitive diagnosis by ultrasound, serial β-hCG measurements should be followed every 48 hours—in normal pregnancies, β-hCG level should increase by 66% or greater every 48 hours
- Transvaginal ultrasound provides definitive evidence of ectopic pregnancy, but is not seen in all cases
    - β-hCG >1500 mIU/mL without a gestational sac visualized on transvaginal ultrasound suggests ectopic pregnancy
- Serum progesterone may be decreased (<5 ng/mL)

Treatment

- If there is suspicion of rupture and signs of instability or acute abdomen are present, the patient should be stabilized and requires immediate exploratory laparotomy
- Consider methotrexate (folic acid antagonist that inhibits dihydrofolic acid reductase) if the ectopic pregnancy is unruptured and ultrasound reveals a mass <3.5 cm
    - Dose is calculated according to body surface area and administered in a single dose
    - With single-dose regimen, β-hCG should decline by at least 15% from day 4 to day 7
- Exploratory laparoscopy with salpingostomy or salpingectomy is indicated if medical management is not appropriate, if the patient rejects medical management, or in stable patients with suspicion of rupture
- Regardless of medical vs surgical management, weekly follow-up blood tests are necessary until β-hCG becomes undetectable

Prognosis/Complications

- Success rate of medical therapy is 84% for a single-dose regimen
- Laparoscopic procedures are 95% successful in eliminating the pregnancy
- Risk of recurrent ectopic pregnancy is 10–25%
- Current evidence does not show a clear difference in fertility rates following laparoscopy vs medical management
    - Following surgery, the best available evidence reveals that 86% of women had patent oviducts; in another study, 66% of women who were followed subsequently became pregnant and 23% of those pregnancies were ectopic
    - Following methotrexate therapy, 71% of patients subsequently became pregnant

86. Hyperemesis Gravidarum

Etiology/Pathophysiology

- Hyperemesis gravidarum is defined as vomiting during pregnancy that is severe enough to produce weight loss, dehydration, acid-base disturbances, ketonuria, and electrolyte imbalances, especially hypokalemia
- The etiology of hyperemesis gravidarum is unknown; hypotheses include
  - Hormonal levels: The incidence correlates with the steep rise of β-hCG, estradiol, and progestins between 10–20 weeks gestation; however, little specific evidence directly links these
  - Serotonin plays an important part in the vomiting reflex; however, no specific link to hyperemesis gravidarum has been shown
  - Upper gastrointestinal dysmotility: Progestins cause relaxation of intestinal smooth muscle, resulting in decreased gastric motility; however, the evidence for an increase in gastric emptying time (above that in women without hyperemesis gravidarum) is weak
  - *Helicobacter pylori* infection: Women with hyperemesis gravidarum have higher *H. pylori* infection rates; vomiting improved after antibiotic therapy
  - Hepatic abnormalities: Elevations in LFTs occur more frequently in patients with hyperemesis gravidarum, but this may be a secondary change
  - Nutritional: Evidence of deficit in B_6 levels

Differential Dx

- Molar pregnancy, twins
- Hyperthyroidism
- Drug side effects
- GI disorders (e.g., fatty liver of pregnancy, hepatitis, pancreatitis, peptic ulcer disease, gastroenteritis)
- GU disorders (e.g., pyelonephritis, ovarian torsion)
- Neurologic (e.g., CNS lesions, migraine, pseudotumor, vestibular disease, conversion disorder)
- Diabetic ketoacidosis

Presentation

- Patients typically present between the fourth and tenth week of gestation, with resolution by the 20th week
- Typical presentation includes nausea, vomiting, and weight loss
- Patients usually have evidence of dehydration, including orthostatic hypotension, increased urine specific gravity, ketonuria, and increased BUN and hematocrit

Diagnosis/Evaluation

- Rule out other disorders listed above
- Evaluation includes:
  - Blood pressure and heart rate to assess hydration
  - Assessments of In's & Out's and daily weights
  - Pelvic ultrasound to document pregnancy viability, number of fetuses, and rule out molar pregnancy
  - Abdominal ultrasound and/or upper endoscopy if suspect a GI disorder
  - Laboratory studies include CBC, electrolytes, liver function tests, thyroid function tests, and urinalysis
- Hyponatremia, hypokalemia, and hypochloremia are found in 15–25% of patients
- Elevated ALT/AST and total bilirubin may be found in 15–50% of patients
- Elevated T_4 with suppressed TSH are found in up to 60% of patients
- Less frequent findings include elevated salivary amylase and decreased serum vitamin B_6

Treatment

- Initial treatment includes IV hydration with correction of electrolyte imbalances, strict In's/Out's, daily weights; initial diet include fluids, gradually building to small carbohydrate meals with avoidance of fatty foods; ginger has been shown to improve symptoms
- Some patients benefit from hypnosis
- Vitamin supplementation (B_6 and thiamine)
- Anti-emetics (e.g., meclizine, metoclopramide, dimethydrinate, diphenhydramine, ondansteron, promethazine, hydroxyzine, trimethobenzamine, droperidol); none have been shown to be superior
- Short course of oral methylprednisone for 3 days, followed by a 2 week taper
- Some patients require feeding by nasogastric tube, PEG placement, or parenteral nutrition
- Triple antibiotic treatment of *H. pylori* infection

Prognosis/Complications

- Due to electrolyte monitoring, hyperemesis gravidarum is no longer a fatal disease
- Maternal complications include Wernicke's encephalopathy (confusion, gait ataxia, ophthalmoplegia, convulsions—usually due to malnutrition); diagnosed by MRI
- Central pontine myelinolysis due to overly rapid correction of sodium
- Esophageal rupture secondary to emesis
- Fetal outcome
  - There is some evidence that patients with severe hyperemesis (weight loss of >5% of prepregnancy weight) were found to have smaller infants (<10th percentile)
  - However, other studies have not confirmed this, and it is generally accepted that fetal outcomes are good

87. Gestational Hypertension & Pre-eclampsia

Etiology/Pathophysiology

- Hypertensive disorders occurring in pregnancy include gestational hypertension, pre-eclampsia, and eclampsia
- Gestational hypertension is defined as elevated blood pressure (>140/90) without proteinuria, developing after 20 weeks gestation
- Pre-eclampsia is a syndrome of elevated blood pressure (>140/90), proteinuria, and edema, that occurs in 5–8% of pregnancies (risk factors include first pregnancy, multifetal gestations, underlying hypertension, diabetes, vascular/connective tissue disease, nephropathy, obesity, black race, antiphospholipid Ab syndrome, age >35, genetics, molar pregnancy)
- Eclampsia is defined as the presence of new-onset grand mal seizures in a woman with pre-eclampsia
- Pathophysiology of these disorders involves abnormal invasion of placental cells into the uterine spiral arterioles, leading to endothelial cell dysfunction and vascular reactivity; this abnormal placentation may be secondary to a lack of immunologic tolerance of the maternal cells to the foreign placental cells; activation of the coagulation cascade and loss of vascular integrity (or capillary leakiness); vasospasm and subsequent hemoconcentration are associated with contraction of the intravascular space

Differential Dx

- Chronic hypertension
- Gestational hypertension
- Lupus exacerbation
- Acute fatty liver of pregnancy
- Autoimmune thrombocytopenia or thrombotic thrombocytopenic purpura
- Viral hepatitis
- Exacerbation of an underlying renal disease
- Hemolytic-uremic syndrome

Presentation

- Gestational hypertension: Isolated hypertension (>140/90) that develops after 20 weeks gestation without other signs/symptoms of pre-eclampsia
- Pre-eclampsia: Classic triad of hypertension (>140/90), edema, and proteinuria
  - Other signs and symptoms may include visual disturbances, headache, and epigastric pain
  - Severe cases may include HELLP syndrome (hemolysis, elevated liver function tests, and low platelets)
- Eclampsia: Grand mal seizures that occur during pregnancy, not attributable to epilepsy

Diagnosis/Evaluation

- Gestational hypertension: Blood pressure >140/90 beyond 20 weeks gestation, with no signs or symptoms of pre-eclampsia
- Pre-eclampsia: Blood pressure >140/90 on two separate occasions and proteinuria >300 mg/24 hour urine collection
- Severe pre-eclampsia: Blood pressure >160 systolic or 110 diastolic on two occasions at least 6 hours apart; proteinuria of 5+ gm in a 24-hour urine specimen or 3+ on two random urine samples collected at least 4 hours apart; oliguria (<500 mL in 24 hours); cerebral/visual disturbances; pulmonary edema or cyanosis; epigastric or RUQ pain; impaired liver function; thrombocytopenia; fetal growth restriction
- HELLP syndrome: Evidence of intravascular hemolysis, liver function test abnormalities, and thrombocytopenia
- Laboratory/radiologic evaluation should include CBC with platelets, liver function tests, BUN/creatinine, fetal ultrasound, and non-stress test to assess growth and fetal status
- Eclampsia: Pre-eclampsia criteria plus seizures

Treatment

- The definitive treatment of pre-eclampsia and eclampsia is delivery; timing depends on the severity of disease and gestational age
- Pre-eclampsia of any degree beyond 38 weeks gestation is treated by delivery (either induction of labor or cesarean section when indicated for obstetric reasons)
- Mild pre-eclampsia prior to 38 weeks is treated by bed rest and frequent maternal and fetal surveillance; deliver at 38 weeks, upon documentation of fetal lung maturity, or if disease worsens or complications occur
- Patients with HELLP syndrome or eclampsia must be immediately delivered regardless of gestational age
- There may be some role for careful delay of delivery if severe pre-eclampsia and immature fetus (<32 weeks)
- Administer IV magnesium for seizure prophylaxis during the peri- and postpartum periods
- Stabilize blood pressure with antihypertensives (e.g., hydralazine) when necessary

Prognosis/Complications

- Maternal mortality is ~1% of all women with pre-eclampsia and as high as 20% of women with eclampsia
- Maternal complications include pulmonary edema, hepatocellular necrosis and subcapsular hemorrhage, cerebral edema or hemorrhage, retinal detachment, DIC, postoperative bleeding, delayed wound healing, and abruptio placentae
- Fetal mortality is 4–20%, often due to prematurity, growth restriction, or abruption
- Recurrence in second pregnancy: 20% for mild, 25% severe, and 1–2% eclampsia; patients with HELLP have increased risk of pre-eclampsia in next pregnancy
- There may be an increase in maternal risk of hypertension or diabetes later in life

88. Cervical Incompetence

Etiology/Pathophysiology

- Incompetent cervix is defined as gradual, painless dilatation and effacement of the cervix
- Often occurs during the second trimester of pregnancy
- Estimated to cause 15% of all second trimester pregnancy losses
- Risk factors include previous surgery of the cervix (e.g., dilatation and curettage, conization, cauterization, LEEP), traumatic deliveries resulting in cervical tears (including women with long labors that culminate in cesarean sections), inutero DES exposure, and other congenital abnormalities (women with greater smooth muscle-to-collagen ratio of their cervical tissue may be more susceptible to cervical incompetence)

Differential Dx

- Preterm labor
- Any cause of repeated pregnancy loss
    - Abruptio placentae
    - Infection
    - Uterine anomalies
    - Hormone abnormality
    - Chromosomal abnormality

Presentation

- Classic presentation includes painless dilation of cervix, amniotic sac bulging through a partially dilated cervix in the absence of contractions, bleeding, infection, and/or rupture of membranes
- More common presentation includes cramping, contractions, or bleeding (may be confused with preterm labor)
- Infection, vaginal discharge, and rupture of membranes may occur secondary to an incompetent cervix, further complicating the clinical picture
- Patients may present with a history of second trimester pregnancy loss

Diagnosis/Evaluation

- Clinical diagnosis by routine exam that reveals a dilated cervix with bulging membranes
    - Clinical presentation may be complicated by cramping or contractions; in this setting, history should assess for history of cervical surgery, trauma, or previous pregnancy losses, particularly if at progressively earlier gestational ages
    - Digital examination of the cervix and diagnosis of cervical incompetence in the nonpregnant state have been shown to be of limited usefulness in predicting cervical incompetence
- In patients with risk factors, cervical length can be measured by ultrasound and used as a predictor of cervical incompetence
    - Shortening of the cervix or funneling of the membranes into the internal os has been shown to be an indicator of cervical incompetence

Treatment

- Cervical cerclage is the treatment of choice
    - Cerclage may be placed prophylactically in patients with a history of a prior incompetent cervix
    - Placement should be done at the end of the first trimester, as there is a lower risk of miscarriage
    - Cerclage is contraindicated if rupture of membranes, vaginal bleeding, or contractions are present
    - Vaginal cerclage placement under regional anesthesia is most common
    - Rarely, cerclages are placed abdominally to achieve a more proximal placement or if there is insufficient cervical tissue to place vaginally
- Emergent (salvage) cerclage can be placed after cervical shortening or membrane funneling has been found on ultrasound or examination; however, this is less effective than prophylactic cerclage
- Bed rest, pessaries, and pharmacologic agents are occasionally used, but without proven benefit

Prognosis/Complications

- Patients with prior history of pregnancy loss due to cervical incompetence have a high risk of subsequent pregnancy loss, often at earlier gestational ages
- Prophylactic cerclage placement may be 80–90% successful in preventing premature delivery in patients with a classic history of cervical incompetence; the success rate is lower in patients with a history of preterm deliveries and uncommon presentations
- Cerclage should be removed upon fetal maturity (37 weeks gestation), rupture of membranes, or onset of labor in order to prevent chorioamnionitis, cervical lacerations, or uterine rupture

89. Uterine Rupture

Etiology/Pathophysiology

- Uterine rupture is a nonsurgical disruption of all uterine layers, which usually occurs at a weakened region
- The most frequent cause is uterine scar separation from previous cesarean delivery, which can involve rupture of the fetal membranes, with all or part of the fetus extruded into the peritoneal cavity
    - Classic incision and T-shaped incision carry a 4–9% risk of rupture, low vertical incision has 1–7% risk of rupture, and low transverse has 0.2–1.5%
- Areas of weakness in the uterine wall may be caused by
    - Previous procedures and scarring such as myomectomy or cesarean delivery
    - Overextension of the uterus as in multiple pregnancy or polyhydramnios
    - Structural abnormalities such as a bicornuate uterus or fibroids
    - Abnormal placentation such as placenta accreta
- Other risk factors include maternal age >30, fetal weight >4000 gm, induction of labor, use of uterotonics, maternal müllerian duct anomalies, grandparity, trial of labor in a non-tertiary care hospital, previous cesarean section for dystocia, and a short interpregnancy interval
- Uterine rupture is associated with a 10–15% maternal mortality

Differential Dx

- Placental abruption
- Ectopic pregnancy
- Labor
- Rupture or torsion of the ovarian cyst or fallopian tube
- Degenerative leiomyoma
- Liver/spleen rupture
- Acute/hemorrhagic pancreatitis
- Acute appendicitis

Presentation

- Rupture usually occurs in the later months of pregnancy or during labor; however, it may also have an earlier presentation
- The most common sign is a fetal heart rate pattern with variable decelerations that may evolve into late decelerations, bradycardia, and loss of fetal heart rate
- Sudden onset of intense abdominal pain
- Vaginal bleeding may occur, ranging from spotting to hemorrhage
- Abnormal abdominal contour
- Hypotension and shock
- Cessation of contractions
- Regression of presenting fetal part; loss of station

Diagnosis/Evaluation

- Uterine rupture is a surgical emergency—presentation is often sufficient for immediate treatment
- Definitive diagnosis is typically made during laparotomy

Treatment

- Treatment for uterine rupture is resuscitation, followed by an emergent laparotomy and cesarean section
- A cesarean hysterectomy may be required, although a primary closure may be possible depending on the type of dehiscence
    - If the dehiscence is confined to the previous uterine incision, a surgical repair is often possible
    - If the dehiscence has extended into the uterine arteries or if bleeding is life threatening, a hysterectomy is often necessary
- Physicians or neonatologists should be immediately available to resuscitate the newborn
- General anesthesia is mandatory for cases with fetal compromise or maternal hemodynamic instability

Prognosis/Complications

- The risk of uterine rupture is increased approximately 3-fold during attempted TOL; this risk is increased with induction of labor or the use of prostaglandins
- Uterine rupture results in a 4% increased risk of postpartum hysterectomy and 5% increased risk of severe anemia
- Fetal/neonatal mortality approaches 5%
- Perinatal fetal mortality and morbidity is highest with complete extrusion into the maternal abdomen or prolonged duration of fetal bradycardia before delivery
- Because there is an increased risk of recurrence after the primary event if the uterus is retained, pregnancy should be discouraged and a TOL should not be undertaken

Fetal Complications of Pregnancy

MARY BETH GORDON, MD
MELODY YEN HOU, MD
HOPE A. RICCIOTTI, MD

Section 8

90. Fetal Vessel Rupture

Etiology/Pathophysiology

- Fetal vessel rupture is usually secondary to a velamentous cord insertion (cord insertion site is at the edge of the placenta) or succenturiate placentation (a satellite cotyledon), which leads to unsupported fetal vessels
- These fetal vessels can rupture upon rupture of membranes or with contractions
- Vasa previa exists when these unsupported fetal vessels cross over the internal cervical os; as labor progresses, these exposed vessels are vulnerable to compression and tearing with membrane rupture
- Vasa previa occurs in 1 out of 1,000–5,000 pregnancies; fetal vessel rupture is a rare event, complicating 0.1–0.8% of pregnancies
- Although vasa previa carries a 50% risk of perinatal mortality, that risk increases to 75% once the membranes are ruptured
- The main risk factor for fetal vessel rupture is multiple gestations: The rate of velamentous insertion is 1% in a singleton gestation, 10% in a twin gestation, and 50% in triplet gestation

Differential Dx

- Placenta previa
- Placental abruption
- Uterine rupture
- Cervical/vaginal lacerations
- Cervicitis
- Cervical/vaginal neoplasms
- Hemorrhoids
- Abdominal/pelvic trauma
- Maternal clotting disorders

Presentation

- Most cases of fetal vessel rupture present with frank vaginal bleeding, often after rupture of membranes
- Acute bleeding is usually associated with acute change in fetal heart rate, initially tachycardia, then bradycardia and sinusoidal variation in fetal heart rate signaling fetal anemia
- In rare cases, the laboring patient may be diagnosed prior to bleeding when the fetal vessels are palpated and recognized through the dilated cervix

Diagnosis/Evaluation

- A high index of suspicion is necessary to make the correct diagnosis; diagnosis, therapy, and delivery must be made quickly to maximize fetal outcome
- Although there is rarely time to conduct the following tests, they may be used if the source of blood is in question
  - The presence of fetal blood can be established by alkali denaturation, which is used in the alum-precipitated toxoid (APT), Ogita, and Loendershoot tests
  - If the cells lyse and the serum turns yellow with alkali addition, the source is maternal
  - If the blood fails to lyse with alkali, the blood is fetal
  - Amniotic fluid reduces the sensitivity of the APT and Loendershoot tests
  - Wright's staining of the blood can also reveal a fetal source if nucleated red blood cells are detected
- Antepartum diagnosis of velamentous insertion of the umbilical cord or a succenturiate placenta can be made by ultrasound; transvaginal ultrasound with color Doppler may be used to investigate a possible vasa previa

Treatment

- When the antepartum diagnosis of a vasa previa is made, careful observation and elective cesarean section upon documented fetal lung maturity can improve prognosis
- Treatment for a ruptured fetal vessel is emergent cesarean delivery
- If viable after delivery, the infant should be aggressively resuscitated; fetal blood may be obtained from the placenta under sterile conditions, filtered, and administered to the infant

Prognosis/Complications

- Because the intravascular volume of the term fetus is very small (<250 mL), prognosis is very poor once the diagnosis of fetal vessel rupture is made
- Antepartum diagnosis of vasa previa greatly improves prognosis since cesarean delivery can be performed prior to the onset of labor

91. Fetal Growth Restriction

Etiology/Pathophysiology

- Defined as estimated fetal weight <10th percentile for gestational age
- The etiology may be of fetal, placental, or maternal origin
- Symmetric growth restriction: Head circumference and abdominal circumference are proportionally small; often related to fetal abnormalities or insults early in gestation
- Asymmetric growth restriction: Head circumference is relatively preserved relative to abdominal circumference; often related to utero-placental insufficiency or insults later in gestation
- Risk factors include maternal chronic hypertension, pre-eclampsia, diabetes mellitus, antiphospholipid antibody syndrome, and chronic renal insufficiency
- Small for gestational age (SGA) is a more general term for a small fetus; this term does not necessarily imply pathology

Differential Dx

- Constitutional small size
- Chromosomal abnormality (e.g., trisomy)
- Genetic syndrome (e.g., cretinism)
- Structural abnormalities (e.g., congenital heart defect resulting in congestive heart failure)
- Infection (e.g., rubella, cytomegalovirus, toxoplasmosis)

Presentation

- Uterine fundal height measurements lag behind expected norms; should be within 2–3 cm of gestational age from 18–30 weeks (although this test has poor sensitivity)
- Decreased fetal movement
- Poor maternal weight gain/nutrition or low prepregnancy weight
- Maternal substance use (e.g., alcohol, tobacco, narcotics, cocaine)
- Intrauterine fetal demise
- Placenta previa, abruption, infarction, or circumvallate

Diagnosis/Evaluation

- Establish gestational age and baseline growth parameters using last menstrual period and ultrasound
- Estimate fetal weight by ultrasound, using biparietal diameter, abdominal circumference, and femur length
  - Fetal weight <10th percentile for gestational age suggests growth restriction
  - Ratio of head-to-abdominal circumference can distinguish symmetric and asymmetric growth; normally growing fetus has HC:AC >1 before 32 weeks, <1 after 34 weeks
  - If gestational age is unknown, femur length-to-AC ratio >23.5 suggests growth restriction
- Oligohydramnios at any age can suggest growth restriction
- Elevated maternal serum alpha fetoprotein (MSAFP) or β-hCG
- Umbilical artery Doppler waveforms may show elevated systolic:diastolic ratio (>2.6) or increased resistive index
- Consider amniocentesis for chromosomal analysis and investigate for possible infectious etiologies

Treatment

- Re-assess fetal growth by serial ultrasounds every 3–4 weeks
- Antepartum fetal testing should include non-stress test, Doppler velocimetry, biophysical profile, and contraction stress test
- If fetus >34 weeks, consider delivery
- If fetus <34 weeks, consider amniocentesis to determine lung maturity
  - Deliver if mature
  - Otherwise, consider a course of steroids to improve lung maturity and protect against intraventricular hemorrhage and death; then deliver
- Place the mother in the left lateral decubitus position to improve fetal oxygenation and nutrition
- Begin intrapartum fetal heart rate monitoring with careful attention to late decelerations (more ominous for asphyxia in fetal growth restriction)

Prognosis/Complications

- Increased risk of intrauterine fetal demise
- Increased rate of cesarean delivery
- Increased risk of asphyxia and meconium aspiration
- 6–10 times increased risk of perinatal death
- Neonatal complications include hypoglycemia, hypothermia, respiratory distress, necrotizing enterocolitis, and polycythemia
- Long-term complications include increased prevalence of poor school function, hypertension, stroke, and coronary artery disease
- Potential for "catch-up" growth postnatally depends on the cause of growth restriction, infant nutrition, and social environment

92. Macrosomia

Etiology/Pathophysiology

- Macrosomia is defined as fetal weight >4,250–4,500 gm (corresponding to >2 standard deviations from the mean at term); large for gestational age (LGA) is defined as >90th percentile for gestational age
- Macrosomia results from overproduction of fetal growth factors, including insulin, insulin-like growth factors, and fibroblast growth factors; maternal endocrinologic factors include heightened insulin resistance and maternal hyperglycemia, increased human placental lactogen (from placenta), cortisol, and prolactin
- Maternal glucose and other nutrients diffuse across the placenta, acting in the fetal circulation to stimulate pancreatic β-cell production of insulin and other growth factors; fetal hyperinsulinemia accelerates fuel use and increases fat storage in insulin-sensitive fetal tissues
- Macrosomia may be due to cellular hyperplasia, generally associated with genetic syndromes, or cellular hypertrophy, which is more likely to be associated with metabolic disturbance
    - Macrosomia due to cellular hyperplasia is associated with increased cancer risk (e.g., leukemia, solid tumors), likely due to increased mitogenic activity

Differential Dx

- Constitutional large size (tall mother, male fetus)
- Genetic syndrome (e.g., Beckwith-Wiedemann)
- Maternal factors
    - Diabetes (pregestational or gestational)
    - Maternal obesity
    - Post-dates pregnancy
    - Advanced maternal age
    - Multiparity
    - Previous macrosomic infant

Presentation

- Uterine fundal height measurements ahead of expected norms; should be within 2–3 cm of gestational age from 18–30 weeks (although this test has poor sensitivity)
- Excessive maternal weight gain
- Maternal diabetes or borderline glucose testing
- Macrosomia is a risk factor for shoulder dystocia during delivery

Diagnosis/Evaluation

- Screening to firmly establish gestational age using last menstrual period and ultrasound at 16–18 weeks; monitor maternal weight gain and uterine fundal height
- Maternal glucose tolerance test at 24–28 weeks can identify insulin resistance and the associated increased risk for macrosomia
- Estimate fetal weight by ultrasound, using biparietal diameter, abdominal circumference, and femur length
    - Abdominal circumference is the best single predictor of macrosomia
    - Estimates of fetal weight for LGA fetuses are not as accurate as for growth restricted fetuses (sensitivity only 60%)
- Routine use of ultrasonographic estimates to identify macrosomia is not recommended; however, an additional ultrasound at 32–34 weeks may be useful to guide management in patients with risk factors

Treatment

- Obese mothers should be counseled to lose weight before pregnancy and limit weight gain in pregnancy to within the recommended norms
- Diabetic mothers require strict glycemic control
- Some experts advocate appropriate management of shoulder dystocia during vaginal delivery as the only necessary intervention
    - There is no evidence that early induction reduces the risk of shoulder dystocia and brachial plexus injury in macrosomic fetuses
- EFW >5000 gm is an absolute indication for cesarean delivery
- Due to the increased risk for shoulder dystocia in diabetic pregnancies, elective cesarean delivery may be indicated
    - There is little evidence that cesarean delivery for nondiabetic pregnancies decreases the risk of shoulder dystocia

Prognosis/Complications

- Obstetric complications include increased rate of cesarean delivery, maternal hemorrhage (due to uterine atony, prolonged labor, and overdistended uterus), maternal perineal trauma, shoulder dystocia, and stillbirth
- Neonatal complications include shoulder dystocia (permanent brachial plexus injury in 10% of dystocias), broken clavicle, hypoglycemia, electrolyte abnormalities
- Other complications in infants of a diabetic mother include cardiac anomalies, respiratory distress, renal vein thrombosis, hyperbilirubinemia, polycythemia
- Excellent long-term prognosis overall
- Rare complications include neoplasia (e.g., leukemia, Wilms' tumor, osteosarcoma, hepatoblastoma)

93. Oligohydramnios

Etiology/Pathophysiology

- Normal amniotic fluid volume is approximately 1 L at 36 weeks and progressively diminishes thereafter
- Oligohydramnios is defined as amniotic fluid level <500 mL
- Amniotic fluid is initially an ultrafiltrate of maternal serum
  - The fetus produces amniotic fluid primarily through urination
  - Amniotic fluid is removed from the total pool primarily through fetal swallowing and intramembranous absorption
- Proposed etiologies of oligohydramnios include decreased perfusion of fetal kidneys with reduced urine production, impaired renal/urinary tract structure or function, and membrane pathology
- Oligohydramnios is usually pathologic, particularly when it develops early in pregnancy
- May also result from premature rupture of membranes

Differential Dx

- Fetal growth restriction
- Fetal hypoxia
- Fetal urinary abnormalities (e.g., renal agenesis, urinary tract dysplasia)
- Membrane defect causing leak
- Maternal medications (e.g., ACE inhibitors, indomethacin)
- Post-dates pregnancy

Presentation

- Uterine fundal height measurements lag behind expected norms; should equal gestational age +/− 2–3 cm from 18–30 weeks, although this test has poor sensitivity (30%)
- Decreased fetal movement
- May be found incidentally on ultrasound or on ultrasound screening for patients with known risk factors
- Often associated with intrauterine growth restriction; on ultrasound, oligohydramnios may be earliest sign of IUGR

Diagnosis/Evaluation

- Amniotic fluid <500 mL at 34 weeks gestation is generally considered oligohydramnios
- Diagnosis is determined by ultrasound
  - Amniotic fluid index (AFI) is calculated by adding the vertical depth of the largest fluid pocket in each of four uterine quadrants
  - Most authorities use an amniotic fluid index <5 cm to define oligohydramnios
  - Alternative diagnostic criteria include vertical measurement of the largest pocket of fluid <2 cm
  - Note that ultrasound determination of oligohydramnios has sensitivity of just 5–10% but specificity of 96–98%
- Dye-dilution test (an invasive modality involving injection of dye into the amniotic cavity) is considered the gold standard for diagnosis of amniotic fluid volume abnormalities, but is not clinically practical
- Doppler velocimetry of the umbilical artery may help identify fetuses at risk for adverse perinatal outcome

Treatment

- Maternal hydration and bedrest increases amniotic fluid volume by increasing the maternal intravascular space
- Amnio-infusion in labor limits cord compression
  - Initiated for fetal heart rate decelerations or thick meconium staining of the amniotic fluid
  - May reduce cesarean section rates
  - Not effective as an antepartum treatment
- If associated with intrauterine growth restriction, consider delivery if fetus >34 weeks
  - If fetus <34 weeks, consider amniocentesis to determine lung maturity, and deliver if mature
  - Otherwise, consider a course of steroids (to improve lung maturity and protect against intraventricular hemorrhage and death), then deliver
- Deliver if associated fetal heart rate abnormalities (e.g., late decelerations from placental insufficiency, variable decelerations from cord compression, non-reactive non-stress test) or other evidence of fetal compromise

Prognosis/Complications

- Obstetric complications
  - Cord compression/fetal distress
  - Abnormal fetal lie
  - Increased meconium concentration
  - Intrauterine fetal demise/stillbirth
  - Increased cesarean delivery rate
- Neonatal complications
  - Low 5-minute Apgar
  - Pulmonary hypoplasia from compression of the thorax and lack of fluid inhaled into air sacs of lung
  - Musculoskeletal (e.g., clubfoot, amputation) and facial deformities due to increased uterine pressure/decreased fluid cushion
  - Prognosis is worst for oligohydramnios that develops early in pregnancy, with mortality approximately 50%

94. Polyhydramnios

Etiology/Pathophysiology

- Defined as excessive amniotic fluid volume (≥2,000 mL)
- Amniotic fluid is an ultrafiltrate of maternal serum
  - Amniotic fluid inflow occurs via the lungs ("breathing") and urination
  - Amniotic fluid outflow is primarily through fetal swallowing and intramembranous absorption
- Etiologies include decreased fetal swallowing (esophageal atresia) and increased fetal urination (CNS defects causing impaired vasopressin secretion or osmotic diuresis due to hyperglycemia in diabetic pregnancies)
- Incidence is approximately 1% of all pregnancies; however, polyhydramnios is not always pathologic (indicates an abnormality in about 50% of cases)

Differential Dx

- Normal pregnancy
- Fetal anomalies
  - CNS abnormalities (e.g., anencephaly, spina bifida)
  - GI tract abnormalities (e.g., esophageal atresia)
  - Non-immune hydrops
  - Chromosomal abnormalities
- Multiple gestation
  - Twin-twin transfusion
- Maternal diabetes

Presentation

- Uterine fundal height greater than dates (uterine distention results from excess amniotic fluid)
- Physical discomfort, dyspnea, edema, and oliguria (results from the pressure of uterine distention on surrounding organs and vessels)
- Symptoms are more severe if polyhydramnios and consequent uterine distention develops acutely

Diagnosis/Evaluation

- Physical exam
  - Palpation reveals an enlarged, tense uterus with fetal parts difficult to feel
  - Auscultation reveals distant fetal heart sounds
- Ultrasound is used to determine the amniotic fluid index (AFI)
  - AFI is calculated by adding the vertical depth of the largest fluid pocket in each of four uterine quadrants
  - An index >24 cm (>95th percentile) suggests polyhydramnios
- Dye-dilution test is considered the gold standard for diagnosis of amniotic fluid volume abnormalities; however, this test is not clinically practical as it is an invasive modality involving injection of dye into the amniotic cavity

Treatment

- Mild-moderate polyhydramnios can be managed expectantly with frequent ultrasounds
- Inpatient observation is indicated in patients with severe symptoms (e.g., dyspnea)
- Therapeutic amniocentesis to remove excess fluid may be used for symptomatic relief
- Indomethacin may decrease amniotic fluid volume by impairing fluid production in the fetal lungs, enhancing intramembranous absorption, and decreasing fetal urine production
- In twin-twin transfusion syndrome, invasive methods of equalizing amniotic fluid volume are under investigation (e.g., amniotic septostomy)
- Bed rest, diuresis, and water/salt restriction have not been shown to be effective

Prognosis/Complications

- Obstetric complications
  - Preterm delivery
  - Premature rupture of membranes
  - Umbilical cord prolapse
  - Placental abruption
  - Uterine atony and postpartum hemorrhage
  - Abnormal fetal lie
  - Meconium staining of amniotic fluid
  - Increased cesarean delivery
- Perinatal complications
  - Perinatal mortality correlates with degree of polyhydramnios and with preterm delivery
  - Most infants born at term without anomalies have a good prognosis
  - Low 5-minute Apgar score
  - Macrosomia

95. Hydrops Fetalis

Etiology/Pathophysiology

- Hydrops fetalis is a syndrome of fluid overload, in which excess fluid accumulates in two or more fetal body compartments
- Immune hydrops results from severe fetal hemolytic anemia
  - Maternal exposure to foreign fetal red blood cell antigens prompts the development of immunoglobulins (IgG)
  - Maternal IgG, now sensitized to fetal RBCs, cross the placenta and bind to fetal RBCs, leading to destruction in the fetal reticulo-endothelial system
  - This severe fetal hemolytic anemia results in hydrops fetalis, characterized by a hyperdynamic state, heart failure, hypoxia-induced capillary leakage, and extramedullary hematopoiesis (termed erythroblastosis fetalis, due to erythroblasts entering the fetal circulation)
- Immune hydrops is most commonly caused by Rh iso-immunization, but may be caused by other foreign red blood cell antigens (e.g., Kell, Duffy)
- Non-immune hydrops fetalis may be caused by conditions that result in severe fetal anemia or heart failure (e.g., heart abnormalities, chromosomal abnormalities, inborn errors of metabolism, parvovirus infection, twin-twin transfusion syndrome)

Differential Dx

- Immune hydrops
  - Iso-immunization from a prior delivery of a fetus with paternally-derived foreign RBC antigens
  - Feto-maternal hemorrhage
  - Prior transfusion
- Non-immune hydrops
  - Chromosome anomalies (35%)
  - Twin-twin transfusion
  - Fetal heart failure
  - Anemia
  - Inborn errors of metabolism
  - Infection

Presentation

- Screening for maternal Rh status and the presence of irregular antibodies should occur at the initial prenatal visit
  - Rh-negative mother with an Rh-positive fetus has risk of developing immune hydrops fetalis
  - 13% of Caucasians, 8% of African-Americans, and 1% of Asians are Rh-negative
  - Mothers with positive antibody titers are at risk for sensitized pregnancies and development of hydrops fetalis
- Infants born with hydrops are edematous, pale, limp, and often have respiratory distress

Diagnosis/Evaluation

- Anti-RBC antibody titers ≥1:16 suggest a sensitized pregnancy with risk of hemolytic disease
- Ultrasound findings suggestive of hydrops include polyhydramnios, enlarged placenta, hepatosplenomegaly, ascites, and/or thickening of the abdominal wall
- Amniocentesis is used to measure amniotic fluid bilirubin level to determine the severity of fetal hemolysis
  - Optical density correlates with intensity of hemolytic disease
  - Liley curves of optical densities are used to depict severity of fetal hemolysis: Zone 1 is mild; zone 3 indicates severe disease requiring transfusion or delivery
- Other techniques to quantify fetal hemolysis include fetal middle cerebral artery Doppler flow (correlates with fetal Hb) and fetal blood sampling (used <26 weeks when Liley curves are inaccurate or if fetal hematologic parameters are required)
- Investigations for non-immune hydrops include evaluation for infection (syphilis, toxoplasmosis, CMV, rubella, parvovirus B-19); ultrasound or fetal echocardiogram to determine cardiac structural abnormalities; amniocentesis for karyotype

Treatment

- Prevent iso-immunization
  - If mother is Rh-negative, administer Rh immune globulin (RhoGAM) at 28 weeks
  - Administer within 72 hours of delivery if infant is Rh+
  - Rh globulin also indicated for elective, threatened, or spontaneous abortions; ectopic or molar pregnancy; amniocentesis; CVS; IUFD; trauma; or external version
- Treatment of sensitized pregnancies (i.e., maternal IgG is high and fetus is Rh+, as identified by paternal testing or amniocentesis)
  - Follow amniotic fluid bilirubin or MCA flow
  - If elevated (defined by gestational age norm), assess for decreased fetal hematocrit by umbilical blood sampling
  - Deliver fetus if HCT <30% and >35 weeks gestation
  - Intrauterine transfusion if HCT <30% and <35 weeks
- Treat underlying causes of non-immune hydrops (e.g., pharmacologic management of cardiac arrhythmia, intrauterine blood transfusions for fetal anemia); consider delivery >24 weeks if euploidy and without heart disease

Prognosis/Complications

- Immune hydrops fetalis
  - 8% mortality for fetus without hydrops
  - 30% mortality for fetus with hydrops
  - Most surviving fetuses have normal neurologic outcomes; however, 10% have developmental delay or cerebral palsy
  - Hearing loss may be a complication of long-term exposure to high bilirubin levels
- Non-immune hydrops fetalis
  - 95% mortality if develops before 24 weeks gestation
  - 80% mortality for fetus >24 weeks without heart disease and with normal ploidy
  - Maternal "mirror syndrome" signifies the development of pre-eclampsia with severe edema (mirrors fetus)
  - Obstetric complications: Preterm labor, postpartum hemorrhage, retained placenta

96. Intrauterine Fetal Demise

Etiology/Pathophysiology

- Fetal death may occur at any time during a pregnancy
- Intrauterine fetal demise (IUFD) is generally defined as fetal death beyond 8 weeks gestation
- Many terms describe fetal death
  - "Miscarriage" is a lay term
  - "Missed abortion" denotes fetal demise and retention within the uterus, diagnosed by ultrasound
  - "Stillbirth" denotes delivery of a dead fetus beyond 20 weeks gestation
- 10–15% of recognized pregnancies end in loss of the fetus
  - 90% of losses occur in first trimester, most due to chromosomal aberrations
  - The incidence of IUFD beyond 20 weeks is 5–10 per 1000 pregnancies
- Pathophysiology of demise includes fetal chromosomal abnormalities, structural abnormalities, and placental abnormalities or maternal diseases that prohibit adequate flow of nutrients (including oxygen) to the fetus or otherwise disrupt normal fetal development
  - Chromosomal losses include monosomy X; trisomy 13, 18, or 21; and sex chromosomal polysomies
  - Autosomal trisomies are the largest class of chromosomal abnormality

Differential Dx

- Fetal causes: Genetic abnormalities, IUGR, infection (e.g., syphilis, parvovirus, toxoplasmosis, listeriosis)
- Maternal causes: Pre-eclampsia, diabetes, hypertension, renal or thyroid disease, anti-phospholipid antibody syndrome, thrombophilias
- Pregnancy-related: Cord accident, abruption, severe oligohydramnios

Presentation

- Early demise often presents as spotting or bleeding
- Third trimester losses present with decreased or absent fetal movement
- Physical exam will reveal absence of uterine growth and no cardiac activity
- Risk factors include
  - Advanced maternal age
  - Previous fetal death
  - Smoking
  - Obesity
  - Low socioeconomic status
  - Elevated maternal serum alpha fetoprotein in the second trimester
  - Abnormal biophysical profile, oligohydramnios, and absent or reversed end diastolic flow in the umbilical artery

Diagnosis/Evaluation

- Ultrasound allows diagnosis of fetal demise before overt clinical signs are evident (absent cardiac activity is diagnostic)
- Pregnancies at risk for IUFD can be followed with the biophysical profile
  - This test is useful to guide management decisions if the fetus has reached viability
  - False negative rate of 0.7/1000
- Patients with recurrent early trimester fetal loss or any stillbirth may be evaluated for etiology to evaluate the risk of recurrence
  - Basic evaluation includes detailed maternal and family medical and obstetric history, maternal anticardiolipin antibody, and lupus anticoagulant
  - If >20 weeks, pathologic exam is recommended, including autopsy; examination of placenta, membranes, and umbilical cord; and karyotype
  - Although appropriate cultures, Kleinhauer-Betke (for maternal-fetal hemorrhage), and antinuclear antibody are often sent, these tests have low yield
- Cytogenetic studies may be done in parents of stillborn fetuses

Treatment

- Prenatal counseling to minimize risk factors
- Optimize management of known maternal disease (e.g., normalize blood pressure and glucose)
- Antenatal surveillance is necessary for high-risk pregnancies with maternal monitoring of fetal movements; formal biophysical profile (fetal movement, tone, "breathing," amniotic fluid volume, and non-stress test) can guide the decision to deliver once fetus is viable
- Uterine evacuation is usually by medical or surgical abortion
  - Dilation and evacuation in fetuses <20 weeks
  - Induction of labor with intravaginal prostaglandins in fetuses >20 weeks
- Administer RhoGAM if Rh-incompatible
- Emotional counseling for parents and family
- Monitor physical exam and labs for maternal complications (e.g., DIC) for a month following demise

Prognosis/Complications

- Women who experience death of a fetus are at increased risk for recurrence
  - The overall risk of fetal loss after one prior loss is approximately 20%
  - After three losses, the overall risk is 30–40%
  - Evaluation of the loss can help risk-stratify patients and guide prenatal counseling
- Maternal complications include DIC (usually occurs 2–4 weeks following delivery), infection (e.g., endometritis, sepsis), and depression

97. Meconium Aspiration

Etiology/Pathophysiology

- Fetal hypoxia, cord compression, or GI maturity can cause a vagally-mediated relaxation of the fetus's anal sphincter, resulting in passage of meconium; fetal "respirations" then allow meconium to enter the oropharynx, which may be aspirated at birth
- Effects of meconium on respiratory function include mechanical "ball-valve" obstruction of airways, leading to air trapping, atelectasis, pneumothorax, V/Q mismatch, inhibition of surfactant production, and chemical pneumonitis
- Meconium aspiration is a marker for fetal asphyxia; chronic asphyxia increases pulmonary vascular resistance, resulting in persistent right-to-left shunting after birth
- Meconium-stained amniotic fluid is found in 5–15% of births; of these, up to 33% will develop meconium aspiration syndrome (MAS)
- Risk factors for MAS include thick meconium, nonreassuring fetal heart rate tracing, meconium below vocal cords, post-dates pregnancy, IUGR, and chorio-amnionitis

Differential Dx

- Respiratory distress syndrome
- Infection (e.g., sepsis, pneumonia)
- Transient tachypnea of the newborn
- Persistent pulmonary hypertension
- Pneumothorax
- Heart failure

Presentation

- Mild: Tachypnea, rales, cyanosis
- Moderate: Grunting, retractions, nasal flaring
- Severe: Profound cyanosis/pallor, irregular gasping respirations, barrel chest

Diagnosis/Evaluation

- Diagnosis is confirmed by the presence of meconium below the cords, as observed on laryngoscopy
- Chest X-ray reveals bilateral, diffuse, patchy infiltrates and air trapping; other possible X-ray findings include atelectasis, pneumothorax, pleural effusions, and cardiomegaly
- Hypoxemia and hypercapnia are often present due to partial obstruction of airways; may lead to pneumothorax
- Combined respiratory and metabolic acidosis secondary to severe hypoxia
- Antepartum tests of fetal well being (e.g., non-stress test, biophysical profile, fetal monitoring) are used to identify uteroplacental insufficiency and fetal hypoxia

Treatment

- Removal of meconium via tracheal suctioning (before initiation of ventilation) is indicated if depressed respirations, HR <100, or poor tone
- Amnio-infusion may be used to dilute the meconium and prevent cord compression in cases of oligohydramnios
- If aspiration has occurred and the infant is in distress, improve oxygenation via humidified O_2, CPAP, mechanical ventilation, and/or extracorporeal membrane oxygenation (ECMO)
  - Mild: Requires <40% oxygen therapy for <48 hours
  - Moderate: Requires >40% oxygen therapy for >48 hours
  - Severe: Requires assisted mechanical ventilation
- Due to the increased risk of infectious complications, pneumothorax, and persistent pulmonary hypertension, affected neonates require broad-spectrum antibiotic coverage and close monitoring of respiratory status, blood pressure, and glucose

Prognosis/Complications

- Results in an increased rate of cesarean deliveries
- MAS is fatal in up to 20% of cases
- Short-term complications include pneumothorax (15–30% of cases), persistent pulmonary hypertension (33% of cases), and the need for mechanical ventilation (up to 50% of cases)
- Long-term complications include asthma, abnormal PFTs, seizures, mental retardation, and cerebral palsy

Labor & Delivery

MELODY YEN HOU, MD
JANET F. McLAREN, MD
NGOC T. PHAN
AMINA PORTER, BS
HOPE A. RICCIOTTI, MD

98. Stages & Mechanisms of Labor

Presentation
• The usual presentation of the fetus to the birth canal is the vertex presentation (95% of all labors), with the occiput of the fetus the lowermost part

Stages of Labor
• Stage I: The interval between the onset of labor and full cervical dilatation
• Stage I is further subdivided into three phases
  –Latent phase: The period between the onset of labor and a point at which a change in the slope of cervical dilatation is noted
  –Phase of maximal dilatation: That period of labor when the rate of cervical dilatation is maximal, which usually begins at 2–3 cm dilatation
  –Deceleration phase: A short phase that follows the acceleration phase and terminates at full cervical dilatation (not all investigators have accepted the validity of a separate deceleration phase)
• Stage II: The interval between full cervical dilatation and the delivery of the infant
• Stage III: The period between the delivery of the infant and delivery of the placenta

Mechanisms of Labor
• The mechanisms of labor, also known as the cardinal movements, refer to the changes in the position of the fetal head during passage through the birth canal
  –Engagement: Descent of the biparietal diameter of the fetal head to a level below the plane of the pelvic inlet (the lowest portion of the occiput is at or below the level of the maternal ischial spines)
  –Descent: The greatest rate of descent is during the deceleration phase of the first stage of labor and during the second stage of labor
  –Flexion: Flexion of the fetal head onto the chest optimizes the presenting diameters of the fetal head to the maternal pelvis
  –Internal rotation: The fetal occiput gradually rotates from its original position (usually transverse) toward the symphysis pubis (occiput anterior), or, less commonly, toward the sacrum (occiput posterior)
  –Extension: Extension occurs after the fetus has descended to the level of the maternal vulva. The fetal head is delivered by extension from the flexed to the extended position, rotating around the symphysis pubis
  –External rotation: After the delivery of the head, the fetus resumes its normal face-forward position with the occiput and spine lying in the same plane
  –Expulsion: The anterior shoulder rotates under the symphysis pubis and the rest of the body is usually delivers quickly

99. Initial Labor & Delivery Evaluation

History
• When a laboring patient is admitted to the hospital, a history should be obtained
  –The present pregnancy, obstetric history, and the standard medical and social history
  –The onset, frequency, duration, intensity, and level of discomfort of uterine contractions
  –Any vaginal bleeding, fluid leaking from the vagina (time of occurrence and amount of fluid), and the level of fetal activity

Physical Examination
• On admission, the examiner should obtain vital signs and conduct a brief, general physical exam
• Abdominal examination to assess the lie, size, presentation, position, and degree of engagement of the fetus using Leopold's maneuvers
• Leopold's maneuvers: The first three maneuvers are performed facing the patient; the fourth maneuver is performed facing away from the patient
  –The first maneuver is to palpate the top of the uterus to assess whether the softer, nodular breech or round, hard, freely movable vertex is in the uterine fundus
  –The second maneuver consists of placing both hands on either side of the abdomen to determine which side contains the fetal back or fetal small parts
  –The third maneuver is performed by grasping the presenting part near the pubic symphysis with one hand to again assess the presentation (breech or vertex) and the degree of engagement, as a freely moveable presenting part is not engaged
  –The fourth maneuver, performed facing away from the patient, involves placing both hands on the lower abdomen with the finger tips pointed toward the symphysis to assess the degree of fetal descent and fetal position by palpating the cephalic prominence

Pelvic Exam
• Unless there is excessive vaginal bleeding or a known history of placenta previa, a sterile vaginal exam is performed
  –Amniotic fluid: If the history suggests rupture of membranes, a sterile speculum is inserted and fluid is obtained from the posterior vaginal fornix. If amniotic fluid is present, it turns nitrazine pH indicator paper from yellow to blue, indicating alkaline pH (the vagina is normally acidic, pH 3–4). If placed and dried on a microscopic slide, it shows a typical ferning pattern
  –Cervix: Consistency (soft, firm, moderate), position (posterior, mid, anterior), effacement (shortening, 0–100%), and dilation (0–10 cm) are assessed
  –Presenting part: The nature of the presenting part and, ideally, its position should be determined
  –Station: The station, describing the degree of descent in relation to the ischial spines, is ascertained; when the presenting part is at the level of the ischial spines, the station is zero. There are two systems of measuring how far above and below the presenting part is. In one, the pelvis is divided into thirds above (-1 to -3) and below (+1 to +3) the level of the ischial spines. The other method uses centimeters (-5 to +5). Either system is effective and both are used widely
  –Pelvic architecture: The examiner should assess the diagonal conjugate (distance from the sacral promontory to the lower margin of the symphysis pubis), ischial spines, pelvic sidewalls, and sacrum for adequacy

Fetal Monitoring
• The fetal heart rate should be checked on admission, particularly after a contraction, and thereafter to identify any pathologic heart rate decelerations. (See *Fetal Heart Rate Monitoring* entry)

Laboratory Studies
• A complete blood count, blood type, and screen (submitted to the lab in the event of a need for cross-matching), and urine evaluation should be obtained on admission

100. Fetal Heart Rate Monitoring

Indications

- The goal of fetal heart rate (FHR) monitoring is to identify FHR patterns associated with such fetal conditions as hypoxia, umbilical cord compression, tachycardia, and acidosis; efficacy is controversial, but fetal monitoring has become a standard of care in the U.S.
- Mean FHR varies between 120–160 bpm; beat-to-beat variability is usually present by 28 weeks, representing interplay between the cardio-inhibitory and cardio-accelerator centers in the fetal brain; absence of variability suggests fetal hypoxia, but may also be due to fetal sleep or narcotics
- FHR accelerations represent an intact central nervous system and an adequately oxygenated fetus; the FHR exhibits a transient slowing when fetal myocardial hypoxia is present
- Early decelerations: A slowing of FHR as a contraction begins due to pressure on the fetal head, resulting in a vagally-mediated reflex slowing
- Variable decelerations: Variable in timing; caused by umbilical cord compression; prolonged or deep variables can result in fetal hypoxia
- Late decelerations: Begin after the contraction is under way; indicate uteroplacental insufficiency and represent direct myocardial depression due to hypoxia

Epidemiology

- Continuous electronic fetal heart rate monitoring was introduced into obstetric practice in the late 1960s
- Today roughly 84% of all live births involve electronic fetal monitoring

Side Effects

- The use of fetal monitors can restrict the laboring patient to the supine position in bed; such restriction of mobility may contribute to more discomfort during labor

Alternative Treatments

- Intermittent auscultation by fetoscope is a more basic form of fetal heart rate monitoring; it is conducted every 15 minutes during the first stage of labor and every 5 minutes during the second stage
- Electronic fetal monitoring determines the fetal heart rate and generates a beat-to-beat graphical recording that is correlated with the timing of uterine contractions; it is conducted using either a noninvasive external Doppler technique (most commonly used) or an invasive, more accurate, internal technique that requires placing an electrode on the fetal scalp
- Ancillary tests that can be used if there is a nonreassuring FHR pattern in order to determine if the fetus is becoming acidotic include
  –Fetal scalp stimulation: Confirms the absence of acidosis if stimulating the fetal vertex with a finger elicits a fetal heart rate acceleration
  –Fetal scalp blood sampling: Scalp blood pH <7.20 confirms fetal distress and requires action for delivery

Efficacy

- Several studies have suggested that continuous electronic fetal monitoring has not been shown to improve the intrapartum fetal death rate or neonatal intensive care admission rates when compared to intermittent auscultation
  –The intrapartum fetal death rate using either modality is approximately 0.5/1000 live births
- Neither continuous nor intermittent fetal heart rate monitoring has been shown to reduce the risk of cerebral palsy or long-term neurologic impairment

Complications

- Continuous electronic fetal monitoring has been associated with higher rates of cesarean deliveries without an associated neonatal benefit
- Invasive techniques (internal electrode fetal monitoring, fetal scalp stimulation, fetal scalp blood sampling) carry an increased risk of infection; fetal scalp electrodes and blood sampling should be avoided in the presence of HIV to decrease risk of vertical transmission to the fetus

101. Obstetrical Anesthesia

Indications

- Anesthesia and analgesia for obstetrics includes general anesthesia, regional anesthesia, local anesthesia, and systemic opiates; pain relief can be safely administered and should be made available to all women experiencing pain
- Regional analgesia/anesthesia uses local anesthetics to provide sensory and some motor blockade over a specific region of the body; in obstetrics, regional techniques include spinal and epidural anesthesia, as well as minor blocks (e.g., paracervical, pudendal, and local infiltration)
- Pain during the first stage of labor results from cervical dilation and uterine contractions; painful sensations travel from the uterus via sympathetic nerves through thoracic spinal nerves T10, T11, T12; pain during the second stage of labor results from distention of the pelvic floor, vagina, and perineum by the presenting part of the fetus through sacral nerves S2, S3, S4 (pudendal nerve)
- Some women prefer nonpharmacologic methods of pain control, including breathing techniques, warm baths, massage, partner coaching, and education
- Analgesia is important for women with certain medical conditions (especially cardiac disorders), obstetrical manipulations (breech, multiple pregnancies), perineal laceration repair, C-section, and manual extraction of the placenta
- General anesthesia should be immediately available in emergency laparotomy

Epidemiology

- Epidural anesthesia is the most common method of pain relief during labor used in the U.S.

Side Effects

- Systemic opiate administration can cause respiratory depression (in both mother and newborn), nausea and vomiting, and over-sedation
- Spinal and epidural analgesia may cause maternal hypotension, impaired ambulation, voiding inability, nausea/vomiting, and pruritis
- Some studies suggest that epidural analgesia decreases the rate of cervical dilation in the first stage of labor and reduces the ability to push during the second stage; recent reports have not found an adverse effect on progress of labor when lower concentrations of anesthetic are used

Alternative Treatments

- Local analgesia is used primarily in laceration or episiotomy repair and involves infiltration of the analgesic agent (bupivacaine, lidocaine, or chloroprocaine) at the wound site
- Systemic analgesia with opioids provides moderate pain relief and sedation; all freely cross the placenta
- Regional analgesia refers to spinal sensory nerve blockade through a number of techniques: Lumbar epidural analgesia is most commonly used and involves the continuous injection of local anesthetic and/or opioid agents into the epidural space; spinal analgesia involves one injection into the subarachnoid space, which works rapidly but lasts for only 1–2 hours (often used for cesarean sections); the combined spinal-epidural technique (CSE) combines the advantages of both; paracervical blockade is useful at the end of the first stage of labor; and pudendal nerve blockade by local infiltration of the nerve is often useful in the second stage
- General anesthesia is usually used for emergency cesarean section, breech head entrapment, or instrumentation (e.g., postpartum D & C for retained placenta)

Efficacy

- Epidural analgesia is consistently more effective than opioid analgesia for pain relief
- Studies have found no difference in cesarean delivery rates or Apgar scores, and minimal differences in neurologic and behavioral outcomes in epidural-exposed vs opioid-exposed infants

Complications

- Complications of epidural use include back pain, maternal hypotension (up to 10%) which can lead to fetal bradycardia; dural puncture (1–3%) resulting in high spinal drug levels or postdural puncture headache (1–3%); epidural hematoma (<1%); nerve injury or paralysis is rare (<0.06%); there is controversy as to whether epidural use increases forceps and cesarean delivery, but most recent studies do not confirm this
- Narcotics may cause respiratory depression in newborns, requiring mechanical ventilation and administration of naloxone
- General anesthesia carries an increased risk of aspiration, which can result in aspiration pneumonitis; it also increases the risk of postpartum hemorrhage due to uterine relaxation

102. Induction of Labor

Indications

- The goal of induction of labor is to stimulate contractions to achieve vaginal delivery before the spontaneous onset of labor; if the cervix is unfavorable for delivery, agents may be used for cervical ripening
- Indications for induction of labor include abruptio placentae, chorio-amnionitis, fetal demise, premature rupture of membranes, post-term pregnancy, maternal medical conditions (diabetes mellitus, renal disease, chronic pulmonary disease, chronic hypertension), fetal compromise (growth restriction, iso-immunization), pre-eclampsia or eclampsia, and logistics (history of rapid labor, distance from obstetrical facility, weather conditions)
- The status of the cervix can be determined by the Bishop score: 0–1 points are given for dilation, effacement, station, consistency, and position
- Oxytocin is an octapeptide that stimulates labor; uterine response occurs after 3–5 minutes and steady state is reached after 40 minutes; there is a gradual increase in response from 20–30 weeks; cervical dilation, parity, and gestational age are predictors of dose response for labor stimulation
- Before induction one must confirm gestational age; fetal lung maturity assessment should be done when <39 weeks and no medical need for induction

Epidemiology

- The overall rate of induction of labor in the U.S. has increased from 90/1000 live births in 1980 to 184/1000 live births in 1997

Side Effects

- Prostaglandin E2 (dinoprostone) should be avoided in women with asthma, as it can cause bronchospasm (paradoxically, prostaglandin E2 is a bronchodilator); also avoid in those with renal or liver disease
- Prostaglandin E1 (misoprostol) has a higher risk of meconium passage than prostaglandin E2
- Uterine hyperstimulation (contractions lasting 2 or more minutes, or more than five contractions in 10 minutes) may occur with the use of PGE analogs
- Uncommon maternal side effects from PGE include fever, vomiting, diarrhea

Alternative Treatments

- Pharmacologic agents
    - Prostaglandin E2 (dinoprostone): Gel or vaginal insert
    - Prostaglandin E1 (misoprostol): Oral or vaginal insert
    - Mifepristone (RU-486): Not widely used currently
- Mechanical techniques
    - Membrane stripping: Weekly finger sweeping
    - Amniotomy or artificial rupture of membranes (AROM)
    - Balloon (Foley) catheter inserted above cervical os +/- extra-amniotic saline infusion
    - Hygroscopic cervical dilators
- Oxytocin: IV oxytocin stimulates uterine contractions
    - Infusion protocols include low dose, high dose, continuous, and pulsatile
    - The dose is increased until normal progression of labor or uterine pressure of 150–350 Montevideo units
    - Maximum dose usually 40 mU
    - Monitor uterine activity and fetal heart rate for signs of uterine hyperstimulation (≥5 contractions in 10 minutes) with or without signs of fetal distress

Efficacy

- Cervical exam: Bishop's score ≥6 predicts successful induction; Bishop's score <6 pre-induction suggests that cervical ripening is needed and increases the risk of failed induction
- PGE2 (dinoprostone) is superior to placebo in promoting cervical ripening; PGE1 (misoprostol) is a newer method and has recently been shown to be either superior or as efficacious as PGE2
- The cesarean delivery rate has been reported to be higher with PGE2 (dinoprostone) compared with PGE1 (misoprostol); however, further study is needed
- Contraindications to induction include transverse lie; transfundal uterine surgery; certain fetal anomalies (severe hydrocephalus, omphalocele containing liver); and fetal distress

Complications

- Induction or augmentation of labor is contraindicated with prior uterine classic incision; risk of uterine rupture or scar dehiscence is 5–8%
- Use of misoprostol (PGE1) in women with prior lower segment cesarean increases the risk of uterine rupture
- Uterine hyperstimulation is increased with higher doses of prostaglandins; with non-reassuring fetal heart rate patterns and no response to corrective measures (maternal repositioning and supplemental oxygen), cesarean delivery is indicated

103. Dystocia & the Augmentation of Labor

Etiology/Pathophysiology

- Dystocia is defined as difficult labor; may result from abnormalities involving the cervix, uterus, fetus, maternal pelvis, or a combination of these
- Augmentation of labor is the amplification of normal, spontaneous contractions; indicated when there is failure to progress labor due to uterine contractions that are inadequate to produce cervical change or fetal descent
- Abnormal labor may be classified as either slower-than-normal (protraction disorders) or complete cessation of progress (arrest disorder)
- Abnormalities of the first stage of labor complicate 8–11% of all cephalic deliveries; second-stage abnormalities are equally common
- Identification of abnormal labor requires assessment of the *powers* (uterine contractility), the *passenger* (fetus), and the *passage* (the pelvis)
- The first stage of labor has been divided into a latent and active phase; during the latent phase, uterine contractions are infrequent and irregular and result in modest discomfort, and there is gradual effacement and dilation of the cervix; the active phase is characterized by an increased rate of cervical dilation (signaled by an abrupt change in the slope of the curve that results when cervical dilation is plotted against time), which occurs when the cervix reaches 3–4 cm

Differential Dx

- Latent phase of labor
- False labor

Presentation

- Abnormal labor patterns of dilation are progress <1.2 cm/hr in a nulligravida and <1.5 cm/hr in a multipara
- Abnormal labor patterns of descent are progress <1.0 cm/hr in a nulligravida and <2.0 cm/hr in a multipara
- Arrest of dilation is defined as >2 hours (in both nulligravidas and multiparas) with no cervical change
- Arrest of descent is defined as >1 hour (in both nulligravidas and multiparas) with no descent

Diagnosis/Evaluation

- Assessment of *powers* during the active phase of the first stage of labor involves investigation of uterine contractility; the minimal contractile pattern of 95% of women in spontaneous labor consists of 3–5 contractions in a 10 minute window; it may be quantified by palpation, external tocodynamometry, or internal uterine pressure sensors
- Before an arrest disorder can be diagnosed, the following criteria should be met: 1) the latent phase is completed (cervical dilation is a minimum of 4 cm); and 2) a uterine contraction pattern exceeds 200 Montevideo units (the strength of contractions in millimeters of mercury multiplied by frequency per 10 minutes) for 2 hours
- Assessment of the *passenger* (the fetus) consists of estimating fetal weight, position, and attitude
- Assessment of the *passage* is done through clinical pelvimetry to identify the general architectural features of the pelvis

Treatment

- Amniotomy is commonly used to augment labor; when performed at 4–6 cm cervical, it may shorten the active phase and decrease the need for oxytocin augmentation
- Oxytocin is used to effect uterine activity to produce cervical change or fetal descent; its half-life is 3–5 minutes (allowing uterine hyperstimulation to resolve with discontinuation of the oxytocin); the response to oxytocin depends on pre-existing uterine activity or sensitivity, gestational age, and cervical status
- A system of labor management, termed active management of labor, includes strict criteria for the diagnosis of labor, early amniotomy, hourly vaginal exams, high-dose oxytocin if progress is not at least 1 cm of dilation since last exam, and strict criteria for the interpretation of fetal compromise

Prognosis/Complications

- Contraindications to augmentation are similar to those for labor induction and may include placenta or vasa previa, umbilical cord presentation, prior classic uterine incision, active genital herpes infection, pelvic structural deformities, or invasive cervical cancer
- With amniotomy, there is a greater number of variable decelerations but the incidence of severe abnormal fetal heart rate patterns or operative intervention is not increased
- Adverse effects of oxytocin are primarily dose related; the most common effect is fetal heart rate decelerations associated with uterine hyperstimulation
- Active management of labor may decrease cesarean delivery rates by 4.8%

104. Vaginal & Operative Vaginal Delivery

Indications

- The goals of a normal vaginal delivery are the reduction of trauma to the mother, prevention of injury to the fetus, and initial support of the newborn
- Operative vaginal deliveries are those deliveries that are assisted with a vacuum or forceps: Indicated when shortening of the second stage of labor is in the best interest of the mother or fetus; specific indications include nonreassuring fetal heart rate, underlying maternal medical disorders that restrict the safety of pushing efforts (e.g., cardiac disease, unstable neurovascular abnormalities), prolonged second stage of labor, and maternal exhaustion
- Most authorities consider vacuum extraction inappropriate before 34 weeks gestation due to the risk of fetal intraventricular hemorrhage
- Operative vaginal delivery (vacuum or forceps) is contraindicated if the fetus is known to have a bone demineralization condition (e.g., osteogenesis imperfecta) or a bleeding disorder (e.g., allo-immune thrombocytopenia, hemophilia, von Willebrand's disease)

Epidemiology

- Studies before 1970 suggested that fetal morbidity/mortality increased when the second stage of labor exceeds 2 hours; fetal monitoring now allows identification of fetuses that may not be tolerating labor; thus, the length of second stage is no longer an indication for the operative delivery
- In 1997 in the U.S., 9% of births were assisted by forceps or vacuum

Side Effects

- The risk of shoulder dystocia increases when operative vaginal delivery is used in cases of suspected macrosomia or prolonged labor
- Operative delivery requires adequate maternal anesthesia, either with epidural or pudendal block
- Episiotomy (an incision made in the perineum to facilitate delivery) is used to minimize trauma to the maternal perineum; there is controversy about the efficacy of this procedure, as there may be an associated increase in third- and fourth-degree lacerations

Alternative Treatments

- Expectant management may be an alternative to operative vaginal delivery when fetal status is reassuring
- Outlet forceps: The scalp is visible at the introitus without separating the labia, the fetal skull has reached the pelvic floor, the fetal head is at or on the perineum, and the angle between the anteroposterior line and the sagittal suture does not exceed 45 degrees
- Low forceps: The leading point of the skull is at +2 station or more, subclassified as to whether the angle between the sagittal suture and anteroposterior exceeds 45°
- Mid-forceps: The head is engaged but the presenting part is above station +2
- Cesarean delivery may be an alternative to operative vaginal delivery

Efficacy

- It is not clear if operative delivery decreases cesarean section rates

Complications

- Both forceps delivery and vacuum extraction have been associated with the development of maternal pelvic floor trauma and hematoma
- The incidence of serious complications from vacuum delivery is 5%; may result in scalp lacerations, cephalohematoma, subgaleal hematomas (collections of blood in the potential space between the cranial periosteum and the epicranial aponeurosis); intracranial hemorrhage, retinal hemorrhage, and hyperbilirubinemia (from cephalohematoma)
- Complications from forceps application include bruising on the fetal face and head, lacerations to the fetal head and birth canal, facial nerve palsy, and intracranial damage

105. Episiotomy

Etiology/Pathophysiology

- An episiotomy is a prophylactic incision in the perineum made during the second stage of labor in order to facilitate vaginal delivery
- Episiotomies are performed in >50% of vaginal deliveries
- Complications of pelvic floor trauma were traditionally thought to be reduced by episiotomies; however, current data do not support this tenet: Recent studies show that episiotomy results in weakness of pelvic floor muscle strength, perineal pain, sexual problems, lack of protection against anal sphincter rupture, and urinary incontinence
- Thus, current trends are to avoid prophylactic episiotomy
- Indications for episiotomy include
  - Arrested/protracted descent
  - Instrumental delivery (vacuum or forceps)
  - Expedition of delivery in setting of fetal distress
  - Malpresentation
  - Anticipation/preparation for management of suspected shoulder dystocia
- Benefits of episiotomy include straight surgical incision rather than a ragged tear and reduced length of the second stage of labor

Differential Dx

Presentation

- Midline/median episiotomy
  - Common in U.S.
  - Vertical midline incision from posterior fourchet to rectum
  - 2–3 cm in length
- Mediolateral episiotomy
  - Common in Europe
  - Vertical incision ~45° from inferior portion of hymenal ring
- Rarely, an anterior episiotomy will be performed in women with previous genital mutilation

Diagnosis/Evaluation

- Classification of perineal injuries
  - First-degree tear: Vaginal mucosa only
  - Second-degree tear: Extends to subcutaneous tissue of perineal body
  - Third-degree tear: Extends to external anal sphincter
  - Fourth-degree tear: Extends to rectal mucosa; may lead to incontinence and pelvic prolapse

Treatment

- Suture in layers to prevent hematoma formation
- If damage occurs to the external anal sphincter, perform primary approximation of the episiotomy and direct opposition of external anal sphincter
- If incision is free of hematoma/ecchymosis, perform routine cleansing, Sitz bath, and use NSAIDs for pain relief and swelling
- If incision is mediolateral or there is hematoma formation, ecchymosis, third- or fourth-degree tear
- Urinary catheterization may be needed since peri-urethral swelling may prevent voiding
- Drain any hematoma or infection
- Daily cleansing with Sitz bath

Prognosis/Complications

- Median episiotomy is associated with increased incidence of third- and fourth-degree tears, increased blood loss, especially if extended beyond transverse perineal muscle
- Mediolateral episiotomy is less likely to be associated with damage to the rectum but has poorer cosmetic results and causes greater blood loss than median episiotomy
- Perineal infection following episiotomy is rare; pain is often in excess of findings; treat with incision and drainage and antibiotics

106. Cesarean Section Delivery

Indications

- Cesarean section (C-section) delivery describes the delivery of a fetus through a surgical incision of the anterior uterine wall
- Performed to decrease fetal and maternal morbidity and mortality
- Maternal indications include failure to progress in labor (this is the most common indication for a primary cesarean delivery), failed induction of labor, dystocia, maternal disease (e.g., cardiac disease, diabetes, cervical cancer, HIV, HSV), and elective repeat cesarean section
- Fetal indications include nonreassuring fetal heart rates, fetal malpresentation (transverse lie, breech presentation), uterine cord prolapse, severe macrosomia, fetal bleeding diathesis, some multiple gestations, and some fetal anomalies (e.g., hydrocephalus, open neural tube defects)
- Uteroplacental indications include placenta previa, placental abruption, prior uterine rupture, previous classical cesarean delivery or uterine surgery, and large fibroids or other outlet obstruction

Epidemiology

- Cesarean delivery now accounts for roughly 25% of all deliveries
- It is the most common hospital-based operative procedure in the U.S.

Side Effects

- There is evidence that cesarean delivery increases the risk of abnormal placentation in future pregnancies
  - Women with one prior cesarean delivery are at 2.6 times greater risk of placenta previa in a subsequent pregnancy
  - The risk of placenta accreta (abnormal adherence of the placenta to uterine wall) also increases with the number of prior cesareans
- A "classical" uterine incision is a contraindication for a future trial of labor in a subsequent delivery due to the increased risk of uterine rupture (see *Vaginal Birth After Cesarean Delivery* entry)

Alternative Treatments

- The abdominal skin incision may be transverse or vertical
  - Pfannenstiel incision (low transverse) provides decreased post-operative pain, strong wound closure, and good cosmetic results; however, it requires a longer operative time and may not provide adequate exposure in obese patients
  - A midline vertical incision provides rapid access to the abdominal cavity and optimal exposure but higher rates of wound dehiscence and postoperative pain
- The uterine incision may be transverse or vertical
  - A transverse lower uterine segment hysterotomy (Kerr incision) is used most commonly and is associated with lower blood loss, easier repair, and the possibility of a trial of labor in a subsequent delivery
  - A low vertical (Kronig) or a high vertical (classic) hysterotomy is used in selected cases of lower uterine segment pathology (adhesions, fibroids), a poorly developed lower uterine segment (preterm fetus), anterior placenta previa/accreta, impacted transverse lie, preterm breech, or certain fetal anomalies (severe hydrocephalus)

Efficacy

- Maternal mortality from cesarean delivery is <0.1%; this is higher than for vaginal delivery
- Studies have shown decreased perinatal/neonatal mortality and serious morbidity for breech presentation at term with elective cesarean delivery compared to planned vaginal delivery
- The increase in the national cesarean delivery rate over the last few decades has not appreciably affected the overall perinatal mortality rate

Complications

- Infectious morbidity (despite antibiotic prophylaxis)
- Hemorrhage (1–2% require blood transfusion)
- Injury to pelvic organs
- Thrombo-embolic disease (four-fold increased risk of DVT formation with cesarean compared to vaginal delivery)
- Anesthetic complications
- Fetal risks may include birth trauma and transient tachypnea of the newborn as fetal lung fluid has not yet begun to be reabsorbed or expelled as in vaginal delivery

107. Vaginal Birth After Cesarean Delivery

Indications

- Vaginal birth after cesarean delivery (VBAC) may be attempted safely in carefully selected women who have had a prior cesarean delivery
- The American College of Obstetricians and Gynecologists (ACOG) guidelines recommend the following selection criteria
  - Only one or two previous low-transverse cesarean deliveries
  - Clinically adequate pelvic dimensions for fetal passage
  - No other uterine scars or previous uterine rupture
  - A physician must be immediately available throughout active labor and capable of performing an emergency cesarean delivery, with availability of anesthesia and personnel for emergency cesarean delivery
- Contraindications to VBAC include prior classic or T-shaped uterine incision, prior transfundal myomectomy or other uterine surgery, and contracted pelvis
- Further study is needed to make recommendations for women with more than two prior cesarean deliveries, multiple gestation, unknown uterine scar, low vertical incision, post-term or preterm gestation, or suspected macrosomia

Epidemiology

- VBAC rates rose from 3% in 1981 to a peak of 31% in 1998, but have now decreased to roughly 16%
- This decrease is due to the recognition of the small but significant risk of uterine rupture, with poor outcome for both mother and infant
- Increasingly, these adverse events during trial of labor have led to malpractice suits

Side Effects

- Induction or augmentation of labor with oxytocin is not contraindicated in women undergoing a trial of labor for attempted VBAC; however, uterine rupture rates are higher in prostaglandin-induced labor
- Misoprostol (PGE1) should not be used in patients with previous cesarean delivery or uterine surgery for cervical ripening due to the risk of uterine rupture
- Use of oxytocin or prostaglandin gel requires close patient monitoring; studies suggest prostaglandin gel appears to be safe but there are occasional reports of uterine rupture with these preparations; high infusion rates of oxytocin appear to place women at greater risk

Alternative Treatments

- Pregnant women with a previous cesarean delivery must choose between elective repeat cesarean delivery and a trial of labor for vaginal birth; although the absolute risk of major maternal complications (uterine rupture, hysterectomy, and operative injury) is small, the risks are greater for attempted VBAC than for planned cesarean delivery

Efficacy

- VBAC is successful in 60–80% of trials of labor in selected women; the success rate is highest for women whose previous cesarean was for breech presentation; the success rate is lowest for women for whom dystocia was the indication for their previous cesarean; success rates decrease as the number of prior cesareans increases
- When VBAC is successful, benefits include lower rates of maternal wound infection, postpartum fever, blood transfusion, hysterectomy, thrombo-embolic complications, neonatal respiratory problems, and length of hospital stay

Complications

- The most serious maternal complication is uterine rupture; risk factors include previous classic uterine incision (4–9% risk compared to 0.2–1.5% risk with low transverse incision); maternal age >30 years; fetal weight >4000 gm; induction of labor; previous cesarean delivery for dystocia; and trial of labor in a nontertiary care facility
- Other major complications include operative injury and hysterectomy (0.2% risk) after failed VBAC
- The risk of perinatal death (0.1–0.2%) is higher for women attempting VBAC than for women undergoing planned repeat cesarean delivery, even in the absence of uterine rupture

Complications of Labor & Delivery

MELODY YEN HOU, MD
AMINA PORTER, BS
HOPE A. RICCIOTTI, MD

Section 10

108. Preterm Labor

Etiology/Pathophysiology

- Labor is defined as regular, painful uterine contractions resulting in cervical change; preterm labor (PTL) is defined as labor occurring before 37 weeks
- Preterm birth occurs in 10% of pregnancies in the U.S.; preterm labor with intact membranes accounts for approximately 1/3 of these deliveries; premature rupture of membranes accounts for 1/3; delivery for maternal or fetal indications accounts for remaining 1/3
- Risk factors include preterm premature rupture of membranes, placental abruption, pre-eclampsia or other maternal illness, infection (including UTI), chorio-amnionitis, multiple gestation, uterine anomalies, previous preterm delivery, low socioeconomic status, maternal smoking or cocaine use, low maternal prepregnancy weight, and intra-abdominal surgery
- The strongest predictors of spontaneous preterm birth are the presence of cervicovaginal oncofetal fibronectin, transvaginal sonographic cervical length, an obstetric history of previous preterm birth, and bacterial vaginosis
- The underlying etiology is still unknown, although evidence points to activation of the maternal or fetal hypothalamic-pituitary-adrenal axis, infection, decidual hemorrhage, and/or uterine overdistension

Differential Dx

- Preterm contractions
- Incompetent cervix

Presentation

- Patients may present with intermittent abdominal pain, menstrual-like cramps, lower back pain, pelvic pressure, changes in cervical discharge, or bloody show
- Classically, contractions are felt as rhythmic lower abdominal pains that radiate to the lower back and cause palpable uterine hardening
- However, women in preterm labor may be asymptomatic; in such cases, they may simply present with cervical dilation and effacement

Diagnosis/Evaluation

- A woman subjectively experiencing contractions should be placed on an external tocometer; diagnosis of preterm labor is made by the presence of four contractions in 20 minutes or eight in 60 minutes, with cervical change
- After diagnosis is established, the patient should be evaluated for a precipitating cause (see risk factors above)
- Assess for rupture of membranes (via fern test, nitrazine test, or pooling of fluid in vagina), vaginal bleeding, presentation and station of the fetus, and cervical dilatation and effacement
- Laboratory studies include urinalysis; CBC with differential to assess for infection; toxin screen if indicated; and fibronectin
   - Fibronectin is a substance found in cervicovaginal secretions in early pregnancy and then in the days leading up to labor—in a woman experiencing contractions or in an asymptomatic high-risk gravida, the presence of fibronectin in secretions triples the likelihood of delivery within the following week
- Confirm gestational age from records of early scans, if available, or reassess with ultrasound if necessary

Treatment

- Rehydration is indicated to decrease ADH level, which cross-reacts at oxytocin receptor; rarely effective in advanced PTL
- Tocolytics are agents that decrease uterine contractions; have been shown to delay delivery by 24–48 hours, but have not been shown to reduce premature delivery
   - Tocolytic agents include ritodrine and terbutaline (β-mimetics) and magnesium sulfate (calcium antagonist and membrane stabilizer); other less-often used agents include indomethacin and nifedipine
   - Main goal of tocolysis is to delay delivery 48 hours to administer steroids, so as to enhance fetal lung maturity to decrease the risk of respiratory distress syndrome
- Antibiotics are used to treat infection, ROM, or group B streptococcus prophylaxis; they do not enhance tocolysis
- Deliver if suspect chorio-amnionitis, cervical dilatation of 4–5 cm, nonreassuring FHR, or bleeding suggestive of abruption

Prognosis/Complications

- Up to 50% of women with an episode of PTL go on to deliver at term
- Major morbidity and mortality is from prematurity, which varies according to gestational age and birth weight; survival for infants born at 23 weeks is as low as 30%; 50% survival by 24 weeks; 90% at 30 weeks; by 36 weeks, the mortality rate is similar to that of full-term infants
- Premature infants have an increased risk for necrotizing enterocolitis (NEC), respiratory distress syndrome (RDS), intraventricular hemorrhage (IVH), hypothermia, hypoglycemia, and sepsis
- Preterm infants may have poorer cognitive and behavioral outcomes in the long term
- Magnesium sulfate carries the potential for cardiac and respiratory toxicity

109. Preterm & Premature Rupture of Membranes

Etiology/Pathophysiology

- Premature rupture of membranes (PROM) is defined as leakage of amniotic fluid beginning at least 1 hour before the onset of labor
- Preterm PROM occurs before 37 weeks of gestation
- The fetal membranes consist of an inner layer of amnion and an outer layer of chorion that is directly apposed to maternal decidual tissue
- Infection of the choriodecidual interface often precedes preterm PROM and is thought to play a role in membrane rupture; other risk factors include genital tract infection, low socioeconomic status, uterine overdistension, amniocentesis, second- and third-trimester bleeding, poor nutrition, connective tissue disorders (e.g., Ehlers-Danlos), and maternal smoking
- Organisms may ascend through a short or dilated cervix, or reach the membranes via hematogenous spread; the inflammatory interaction initiates a process that may result in preterm PROM or preterm labor; there is evidence of a common pathway involving matrix metalloproteins and their inhibitors, collagenases, and proteases
- Preterm birth occurs in 10% of pregnancies in the U.S. and PROM is responsible for approximately 1/3 of these births

Differential Dx

- Preterm labor
- Urinary incontinence
- Mucous plug
- Vaginal discharge
- Vaginitis

Presentation

- The most common presentation is a sudden gush of fluid from the vagina followed by a constant, uncontrolled leaking sensation; some patients have small, intermittent leakage or perineal wetness
- Occasionally, a patient may be incidentally found to have decreased fluid volume on ultrasound

Diagnosis/Evaluation

- Assess for fever and tachycardia; abdominal exam should assess for uterine fundal tenderness; fetal monitoring should assess fetal heart rate and uterine contractions
- Pelvic exam should be evaluated by a sterile speculum exam to confirm the presence of amniotic fluid; evaluation includes visualizing pooling of fluid in the posterior fornix, nitrazine paper test to assess pH (amniotic fluid has a neutral pH while the vagina is normally acidic), and microscopic examination for ferning of vaginal fluid on a microscope slide; digital examination should be avoided due to risk of infection
- Laboratory studies include genital cultures for group B streptococcus, gonorrhea, and chlamydia; wet mount evaluation for bacterial vaginosis and *Trichomonas*; CBC with differential to assess for systemic infection
- Ultrasound is indicated to confirm fetal presentation, gestational age, and assess volume of remaining fluid
- Depending on gestational age, consider amniocentesis for fetal pulmonary studies and evaluation for infection (Gram stain, culture, glucose)

Treatment

- Delivery is indicated if suspect amnionitis, fetal distress, vaginal bleeding suggestive of abruption, or substantial cervical dilatation with transverse fetal lie or footling breech presentation (due to risk of cord prolapse)
- Decision to deliver is a risk-benefit ratio
    - The greatest risk of continuing pregnancy is infection (chorio-amnionitis with possible neonatal infection)
    - The greatest risk of delivery is the morbidities associated with prematurity
- Antibiotics decrease the risk of neonatal infection and may increase latency; broad-spectrum IV therapy followed by oral maintenance therapy (often ampicillin/erythromycin) is indicated
- Corticosteroids (to hasten fetal lung development) may be given before 32 weeks, but studies reveal conflicting benefits; they may increase the risk of infection
- There is disputed benefit for short-term tocolysis in order to allow a course of steroids

Prognosis/Complications

- In second-trimester PROM, <50% of women remain pregnant for 1 week; in the third trimester, 80% of women deliver within 1 week
- Noninfectious risks include cord prolapse, abruption (10%), and increased rate of cesarean delivery
- Neonatal infection may occur, resulting in pneumonia, sepsis, or meningitis
- Noninfectious neonatal risks include prematurity, pulmonary hypoplasia (correlates with gestational age at rupture), skeletal abnormalities (from compression)
- 25% maternal risk of chorio-amnionitis (especially with prolonged ROM)
- Fetal demise occurs in 1% of cases (due to cord compression, infection, abruption)

110. Malpresentations

Etiology/Pathophysiology

- Near term or during labor, the fetus normally assumes a vertical orientation (lie) and a cephalic presentation with the fetal vertex flexed (attitude) on the neck—deviation from this norm (5%) constitutes a fetal malpresentation
  - Abnormal fetal lie includes transverse and oblique lie
  - Deflexed attitudes includes face and brow presentation
  - Compound presentation with an upper extremity
  - Breech presentation with complete, footling, or frank breech (see below)
- Malpresentation may result in increased fetal and maternal mortality
- Factors associated with malpresentation include decreased vertical axis of the uterine cavity (as seen in great parity due to laxity of maternal muscular support); structural abnormalities (myomata, synechiae, müllerian duct abnormalities, contracted pelvis); very high or low placental implantation; increased or decreased fetal movement (hydramnios, trisomies, fetal neurologic dysfunction, prematurity); or fetal malformations (hydrocephalus, anencephaly, goiter)
- Breech presentation occurs in 3–4% of term pregnancies, although it is found in 7% of pregnancies at 32 weeks and 25% of pregnancies <28 weeks

Differential Dx

- Transverse lie
- Oblique lie
- Face presentation
- Brow presentation
- Compound presentation
- Breech presentation
- Premature labor
- False labor

Presentation

- Incidental finding by abdominal examination, Leopold maneuvers (maternal abdominal examination to determine fetal position, presentation, and engagement), cervical examination, or ultrasound
- Abnormal progress in labor
- Most face and brow presentations are detected late in labor, often in the second stage

Diagnosis/Evaluation

- Diagnosis of abnormal lie is suspected by abdominal or pelvic examination; ultrasound is used to confirm the lie and rule out major fetal malformations and abnormal placentation
- Face presentation is characterized by full extension of the fetal head; it is palpated through a dilated cervix with the fetal chin chosen as the point of designation; for example, a fetus presenting with the chin in the left posterior quadrant of the maternal pelvic would be called a left mentum posterior
- Brow presentation is characterized by a partially deflexed attitude; the frontal bones are the point of designation
- A compound presentation is found when a fetal extremity is prolapsed beside the fetal vertex
- Breech presentation includes complete (flexed hips and knees), incomplete (incomplete deflexion of one or both knees or hips), and frank (flexed hips and extended knees)

Treatment

- Abnormal lie: Expectant management to wait for spontaneous conversion to vertex if preterm; external cephalic version with subsequent induction of labor or cesarean delivery >37 weeks or once lungs have matured; if ruptured membranes or active labor has commenced, cesarean delivery with possible need for vertical uterine incision to minimize birth trauma
- Malpresentation of the vertex: Carefully monitored vaginal delivery with minimal manipulation may be successful; cesarean delivery if arrest of progress
- Breech presentation: Different categories of breech presentation require different managements; a vaginal delivery may be attempted by an experienced operator with complete or frank breech if carefully monitored, but this remains controversial; external cephalic version is a management option for near-term breech; cesarean delivery is recommended for incomplete or preterm breech

Prognosis/Complications

- Malpresentation increases overall perinatal mortality
- Abnormal lie carries an increased risk of cord prolapse; external cephalic version is successful in 86–96% of cases
- Most infants with face presentation, mentum anterior, will deliver vaginally; persistent mentum posterior makes vaginal delivery less likely, but approximately 20–25% will rotate and deliver vaginally
- Brow presentation carries a higher risk of cephalopelvic disproportion
- Compound presentation carries an 11–20% risk of cord prolapse
- The perinatal morbidity/mortality associated with term breech delivery, when corrected for fetal anomalies, may be higher than elective cesarean; but is controversial

111. Umbilical Cord Prolapse

Etiology/Pathophysiology

- Umbilical cord prolapse occurs when the umbilical cord slips down through the cervix into the vagina
    - Associated with premature rupture of membranes (PROM), a dilated cervix, and an abnormal or inadequately engaged presenting part in the maternal pelvis
    - Conditions associated with an abnormal or inadequately engaged presenting part include fetal malpresentation (breech presentation, particularly footling breech, is associated with a 16–19% risk of cord prolapse)
    - Other conditions that increase the risk of umbilical cord prolapse include prematurity (birth weight <1,250 gm carries 19-fold increased risk), multiple gestations (risk of malpresentation is increased for second-born twin), PROM, multiparity, and polyhydramnios
- Iatrogenic causes of umbilical cord prolapse include artificial rupture of membranes, fetal scalp electrode placement, placement of intrauterine pressure catheter, manual rotation of fetal head, and amnio-infusion/amnioreduction

Differential Dx

- Footling or hand presentation
- Other causes of abrupt-onset fetal bradycardia (e.g., maternal hypotension, placental abruption, uterine rupture, vasa previa)

Presentation

- Umbilical cord is incidentally found on vaginal or speculum exam (a pulsating cord is felt or seen)
- Sudden onset of a prolonged fetal bradycardia or severe variable decelerations after a previously normal tracing and confirmation of the presence of an umbilical cord on vaginal exam

Diagnosis/Evaluation

- When laboring patients have a sudden fetal bradycardia, a vaginal examination should be performed to rule out umbilical cord prolapse
- Patients hospitalized for preterm prolonged rupture of membranes who have abnormal fetal heart monitoring should have a sterile speculum examination to rule out umbilical cord prolapse
- Care should be taken during amniotomy to avoid dislodging the fetal head; an assistant who applies fundal and suprapubic pressure may reduce the risk of cord prolapse; the fetal heart rate should be assessed before and immediately after the procedure

Treatment

- Umbilical cord prolapse is an obstetric emergency; the examiner should attempt to hold up the fetal presenting part so that the umbilical cord is not compressed, as prolonged umbilical cord compression can lead to fetal compromise/hypoxia
- The examiner should leave their hand in the patient's vagina in order to hold up the fetal presenting part while the obstetric team prepares for immediate cesarean section
- In rare cases, the examiner may be able to replace the umbilical cord back into the uterus; this should only be attempted when there is no evidence of fetal compromise

Prognosis/Complications

- Prolonged or unrecognized umbilical cord prolapse may result in fetal hypoxic injury or even death

112. Shoulder Dystocia

Etiology/Pathophysiology

- Shoulder dystocia is an obstetric emergency involving obstruction to the delivery of the fetal shoulder(s) after delivery of the head; it occurs when the anterior shoulder becomes impacted behind the maternal symphysis pubis
- Occurs in 0.2–2% of vaginal deliveries
- Major risk factors are related to fetal weight
  - Fetal macrosomia (birth weight >4,000 gm)
  - Maternal diabetes mellitus, resulting in increased shoulder-to-head ratio and increased incidence of large for gestational age (LGA) infants
- Other associated risk factors include
  - History of prior shoulder dystocia or macrosomic birth
  - Maternal obesity or excessive weight gain during pregnancy
  - Multiparity
  - Operative vaginal delivery (vacuum-assisted or forceps delivery)
  - Abnormal clinical pelvimetry
  - Post-term birth
- The majority of cases occur with no known risk factors; their predictive value is usually not high enough to be clinically useful

Differential Dx

- Labor dystocia or failure to progress due to inadequate uterine contractions
- Fetal abnormality
- Fetal malpresentation

Presentation

- Shoulder dystocia is most often unpredictable and unpreventable
- After a normal labor, gentle traction on the fetal head fails to effect delivery of the shoulders
- The fetal head is delivered but then retracts against the maternal perineum (turtle sign)
- In some studies, labor patterns that show a prolonged active phase of the first stage of labor or a prolonged second stage of labor have predicted shoulder dystocia (however, these data are inconsistent)
- Assisted delivery with vacuum or forceps increases the risk of shoulder dystoria

Diagnosis/Evaluation

- The diagnosis of shoulder dystocia has a subjective component, since the delivering attendant must determine whether ancillary maneuvers are necessary; although severe cases are readily apparent, milder forms may be over- or underdiagnosed
- The diagnosis is made when the fetal head is delivered and then retracts against the maternal perineum (turtle sign) and gentle downward traction fails to deliver the anterior shoulder
- A prolonged or arrested second stage of labor with an estimated fetal weight > 4,500 gm is an indication for cesarean delivery

Treatment

- Shoulder dystocia is an obstetric emergency; the baby should be expeditiously delivered to prevent asphyxia, but without causing brachial plexus injury or fractures
- Initial management steps in sequence should involve
  - Notify appropriate personnel (pediatric staff, anesthesia, nursing)
  - Create space by emptying the bladder and performing a large episiotomy
  - McRoberts maneuver (flexion and abduction of the maternal hips)
  - Moderate suprapubic (not fundal) pressure to disimpact the anterior shoulder
  - Wood's screw maneuver (posterior shoulder is rotated forward and passed under pubic ramus)
  - Delivery of the posterior arm and shoulder
  - Deliberate fracture of the clavicle
  - Cephalic replacement and cesarean section (Zavanelli maneuver)

Prognosis/Complications

- Potential fetal complications include brachial plexus injury (most cases resolve without permanent disability), fracture of the clavicle and/or humerus, hypoxic brain injury, and death (rare)
- Maternal complications may include hemorrhage (11%) and fourth-degree lacerations (3.8%)
- Shoulder dystocia is associated with a recurrence rate of 1–16%
- Planned cesarean delivery to prevent shoulder dystocia may be considered for suspected fetal macrosomia (estimated fetal weights >5,000 gm in women without diabetes and >4,500 gm in women with diabetes)

Postpartum Care & Complications

PHYLLIS L. CARR, MD
JANET F. McLAREN, MD
NGOC T. PHAN
HOPE A. RICCIOTTI, MD
MARION P. RUSSELL, MD

113. Normal Postpartum Care

Etiology/Pathophysiology

- The puerperium is the time period from delivery of placenta to 6 weeks postpartum
- Physical changes that occur immediately postpartum include uterine contraction, uterine involution, and decidual sloughing, resulting in lochia
- Marked leukocytosis occurs during and after labor (leukocyte counts as high as 30,000 per µL can be seen)
- Blood volume returns to nonpregnant levels by 1 week after delivery
- Hypercoagulation occurs due to elevations of plasma fibrinogen and coagulation factors VII, VIII, IX, X
- Decreases in estrogen and progesterone levels after delivery removes the inhibitory influence on lactation and stimulates milk production; the repetitive stimulus of nursing releases prolactin, which stimulates milk production; oxytocin stimulates milk ejection, or "let down," which is initiated by suckling
- There is an immediate weight loss of about 10–13 pounds due to uterine evacuation and normal blood loss, and a further decrease of 4–6 pounds due to diuresis

Differential Dx

- Normal postpartum course
- Maternity blues
- Postpartum depression
- Medical complications, including infection, hemorrhage, and thrombosis

Presentation

- Uterine fundal height immediately postpartum is at the level of 20 weeks size (uterus is slightly below the umbilicus)
- Breast engorgement begins 2–4 days postpartum due to lymphatic and vascular congestion
- Initially as colostrum, milk let-down begins postpartum at days 4–5
- Heavy bleeding associated with sloughing of placenta eschar occurs 7–14 days postpartum
- Lochia persists for 3–8 weeks
- Return of menstruation by 5 weeks in nonlactating mothers and >8 weeks in mothers who are breast-feeding
- 28% of women return to nonpregnant weight by 6 weeks postpartum

Diagnosis/Evaluation

- Postpartum care issues include the establishment of hemostasis, observation of vital signs, and palpation of the uterus for signs of normal involution
- Hospital stay for normal vaginal delivery is 2–3 days; cesarean delivery is 3–4 days
    - Encourage early ambulation to prevent thrombosis
- Patients need not limit physical activity following a normal vaginal delivery; patients should refrain from heavy lifting for 6 weeks after cesarean delivery
- Persistent lethargy requires evaluating for thyroid dysfunction
- Persistent maternity blues beyond 2 weeks postpartum requires evaluation for postpartum depression
- Follow-up visit in 6 weeks postpartum to assess for uterine involution, assessment of mental health, and contraceptive counseling
- Contraindications to breast-feeding include acute hepatitis B, HIV positive, and use of cytotoxic drugs

Treatment

- Pain management with NSAIDs or narcotics
- Infant care teaching
- Breast-feeding support
- Mental health support
- Sexual intercourse may be resumed after 2–3 weeks
    - Contraceptive options include barrier methods (diaphragm, condoms), hormonal methods, and IUD
    - Hormonal contraceptives: Progestin-only methods can be started within 1 week postpartum; combined estrogen/progestin methods may be started 6 weeks postpartum or once breast-feeding is well established (estrogen may decrease lactation)
    - IUDs should be placed after 6 weeks postpartum to avoid uterine perforation or expulsion
    - Diaphragms should be fitted ≥6 weeks postpartum, following uterine involution
    - Sterilization via tubal ligation may be performed immediately following delivery

Prognosis/Complications

- Common complications include infection (e.g., endometritis, mastitis), hemorrhage (e.g., uterine atony), and thrombosis
- Postpartum problems include urinary/fecal incontinence, painful perineum, difficulties with breast-feeding, issues with infant care
- 70% of mothers have "maternity blues" (mild, transient depression) that resolves by postpartum day 10
- 8–20% incidence of postpartum depression
    - Mild to severe (e.g., suicidal ideations)
    - Begins up to 1 year following delivery
    - 20–30% risk of recurrence
    - Treat with counseling and antidepressants
- Postpartum psychosis is rare; occurs from 2–3 days postpartum up to several months; more common in patients with pre-existing psychiatric disorders

114. Postpartum Endometritis

Etiology/Pathophysiology

- Endometritis is defined as inflammation of the lining of the uterus, often due to infection; it primarily involves the site of placental implantation
    - Occurs in 1–3% of vaginal births
    - Occurs in 5–15% of planned cesarean deliveries
    - In cesarean deliveries following extended labor and ruptured membranes, occurs in 15–20% of cases when prophylactic antibiotics are used and 30–35% of cases without prophylactic antibiotics
- Risk factors include cesarean delivery, young age, low socioeconomic status, extended duration of labor with rupture of membranes, and multiple vaginal exams
- Infection is usually polymicrobial and comprised of the normal flora of the genital tract: Group B streptococcus, anaerobic streptococci, aerobic gram-negative bacilli (*E. coli, Klebsiella pneumoniae, Proteus*), anaerobic gram-negative bacilli (*Bacteroides, Prevotella*); *Chlamydia trachomatis* has been implicated in late-onset infections

Differential Dx

- Atelectasis
- Pneumonia
- Cystitis/pyelonephritis
- Wound infection
- Mastitis
- Septic pelvic thrombophlebitis
- Abscess

Presentation

- Fever within 36 hours of delivery
- Tachycardia
- Pelvic/abdominal pain
- Uterine tenderness
- Malaise
- Foul-smelling or purulent lochia
- Can be associated with wound infection

Diagnosis/Evaluation

- Diagnosed is based on clinical presentation
- Laboratory studies include CBC (will show elevated white blood cell count with left shift; keep in mind that leukocytosis normally occurs during and after labor, but there should be no left shift in the absence of infection), urinalysis and culture to rule out urinary cause, chest X-ray in patients with respiratory symptoms, and blood cultures for patients who are immunocompromised or with risk factors for bacterial endocarditis
- Diagnosis can be confirmed with uterine culture, but this is usually not necessary for diagnosis or therapy

Treatment

- Administer IV antibiotics to cover the breadth of organisms in the polymicrobial genital tract flora
    - Acceptable combinations include clindamycin plus gentamicin; clindamycin plus aztreonam; or ampicillin, gentamicin, and metronidazole
    - IV antibiotics should be continued until the patient has been afebrile for 24–48 hours; the usual course of treatment can last 2–10 days depending on the severity of the infection
    - No need for oral antibiotics following IV therapy in uncomplicated cases

Prognosis/Complications

- 90% of patients will improve within 48–72 hours with antibiotic therapy
- Treatment failure is usually due to drug-resistant organisms or other concurrent/complicating infections
- Endometritis may spread to the adnexa, broad ligaments, peritoneal cavity, or pelvic veins
- Complications of endometritis can lead to wound infection in patients with cesarean section, pelvic abscess formation, peritonitis, and septic pelvic thrombophlebitis
- Prophylactic antibiotics for patients with fevers in labor or at the time of cesarean section may be used to prevent endometritis (e.g., first-generation cephalosporin)

115. Postpartum Hemorrhage

Etiology/Pathophysiology

- Postpartum hemorrhage is defined as blood loss >500 mL or a 10% decrease in hematocrit
- A leading cause of maternal mortality; occurs in 10–15% of deliveries, accounting for 28% of maternal deaths in developing countries
- Divided into early (<24 hours) or late (>24 hours) postpartum hemorrhage
  - Causes of early hemorrhage include uterine atony (90%), retained placental fragments (3–4%), cervical and vaginal lacerations (6%), uterine rupture (.0005%), uterine inversion (.0004%), and bleeding disorders (rare); von Willebrand's disease may first present with bleeding problems postpartum
  - Risk factors for uterine atony include overdistension of the uterus (multiple pregnancy, macrosomia, polyhydramnios), multiparity, prolonged labor (especially with oxytocin), amnionitis, and induced labor
  - Causes of late postpartum hemorrhage include subinvolution of the uterus, retained placental fragments, and endometritis
- Effective hemostasis after delivery of the placenta depends upon contraction of the myometrium to compress severed vessels; failure to contract is usually due to myometrial dysfunction or retained placental fragments
- Acute blood loss is the most common cause of hypotension in obstetrics

Differential Dx

- Uterine atony
- Retained placental fragments
- Cervical/vaginal lacerations
- Uterine rupture
- Uterine inversion
- Endometritis
- Vaginal or pelvic hematoma
- DIC
- Bleeding disorder

Presentation

- Bright red blood per vagina
- Hypotension
- Tachycardia
- Shock
- Pelvic pain
- In cases of uterine atony, an atonic boggy uterus may be palpated

Diagnosis/Evaluation

- Visual inspection of the genital tract for lacerations; examination under anesthesia may be necessary for adequate exposure
- Palpation of the uterus to detect uterine atony
- Manual digital exploration of the uterus to detect retained placental fragments; ultrasound may be useful to aid in this diagnosis
- Inspection of the placenta for missing cotyledons
- Laboratory studies include CBC to assess severity of anemia; platelets, PT/PTT, and fibrinogen to evaluate for DIC or consumption coagulopathy; and type and cross

Treatment

- Pharmacologic methods to control uterine bleeding include oxytocin, 15-methyl-$F_{2\alpha}$ prostaglandin, or PGE1
- Volume, blood, and/or clotting factor replacement
- Uterine atony requires manual compression/massage of the uterus and pharmacologic agents to aid in uterine contraction (oxytocin, prostaglandins); proceed to surgical management or embolization if this fails
  - Surgery: Start with ligation of uterine arteries; next proceed with ligation of utero-ovarian artery; finally, proceed to hysterectomy
  - Selective arterial embolization-radiographically guided arterial embolization
- Retained placenta fragments requires manual removal of fragments and curettage; if bleeding is due to abnormal placentation (previa/accreta) and pharmacologic maneuvers fail to correct, proceed with hysterectomy
- Vaginal/cervical lacerations, uterine rupture, and uterine inversion requires surgical intervention

Prognosis/Complications

- Death from postpartum hemorrhage is rare in state-of-the-art hospitals, but more common under less favorable conditions
- Uterine rupture is seen with forceps use, large doses of oxytocin, and vaginal delivery after previous cesarean section
- Other complications include pelvic infection, anemia, transfusion reactions, hepatitis, and renal failure due to prolonged hypotension
- Sheehan syndrome: Acute pituitary necrosis during hypotensive state (intrapartum)
- Asherman syndrome: Secondary amenorrhea due to scarring from uterine curettage

116. Post-Cesarean Wound Infection

Etiology/Pathophysiology

- Cesarean section is the most common surgical procedure in U.S. hospitals
- One of the most common complications of cesarean delivery is infection: Wound infection occurs in 2–5% of women after cesarean section
- Often associated with or preceded by endometritis
- Risk factors
  - Preoperative: Diabetes, obesity, malnutrition, anemia, immunosuppression or corticosteroid use, amnionitis, prolonged ruptured membranes
  - Surgical: Long duration of surgery, poor hemostasis, use of drains, meconium passage
  - Postoperative: Asthma, pulmonary complications and coughing, vomiting
  - Elective cesarean section carries a lower risk than emergent C-section
- The principal causative organisms are *Staphylococcus aureus*, aerobic streptococci, and aerobic and anaerobic bacilli (including group B streptococci, *E. coli, Proteus, Bacteroides*)

Differential Dx

- Endometritis
- Cellulitis
- Seroma
- Hematoma
- Abdominal wall abscess
- Pelvic abscess
- Septic pelvic vein thrombophlebitis
- Mastitis
- Resistant microorganism
- Necrotizing fasciitis

Presentation

- Presentation often includes fever, skin erythema, induration, and tenderness at margins of the incision; purulent drainage may occur from the incision
- Wound infections usually manifest on days 4–7 after cesarean delivery
- Would infection is often preceded by symptomatic endometritis
- The diagnosis of wound infection should always be considered in patients with endometritis who are unresponsive to antibiotic therapy
- Necrotizing fasciitis should be suspected when the margins of a wound are discolored, cyanotic, and devoid of sensation; the subcutaneous tissues easily dissect free of the underlying fascia

Diagnosis/Evaluation

- Wound infection is a clinical diagnosis that is usually made on the basis of inspection of the wound in a febrile patient; when the wound is probed, pus often exudes from the incision; however, some patients may have an extensive cellulitis without harboring frank pus in the incision
- Gram stain and culture of the wound exudate are not routinely needed, because the results of these tests rarely influence the selection of antibiotics or duration of treatment
- A tissue biopsy should be performed and examined by frozen section when necrotizing fasciitis is suspected
- Ultrasound or CT scan may be performed to rule out retained uterine products of conception, hematoma, seroma, or pelvic abscess

Treatment

- Administer broad-spectrum antibiotics and be sure to cover staphylococci
  - Examples include extended spectrum penicillins and first-generation cephalosporins
  - Vancomycin may be used for patients who are allergic to β-lactam antibiotics
  - Antibiotics should be continued until the base of the wound is clean and all signs of cellulitis have resolved
- When pus is present in the incision, the wound must be opened and drained completely and the wound debrided
- Once the wound is opened, a careful inspection should be made to be certain that the fascial layer is intact; if it is disrupted, surgical intervention is necessary to reapproximate the fascia
- Pack wound with wet-to-dry sterile gauze 2–3 times daily
- Once granulation tissue has formed, a primary closure may be performed or the incision may be allowed to heal by secondary intention

Prognosis/Complications

- Fascial dehiscence occurs in 5% of wound infections; this requires a return to the operating room for closure of fascia
- Necrotizing fasciitis is an uncommon but life-threatening complication of abdominal wound infection
  - Rapidly spreading bacterial infection, dissects through body along fascial planes
  - Treat aggressively with antibiotics and surgery
  - Risk factors include diabetes, immunosuppressive disorders, and cancer
- Preventive measures for wound infections include sterile technique, preoperative skin preparation, and prophylactic antibiotics

117. Mastitis

Etiology/Pathophysiology

- Mastitis is a bacterial cellulitis of the interlobular connective tissue of the breast and mammary glands
- Most commonly occurs during the puerperal/lactational period, but may rarely present as a nonpuerperal infection
- Puerperal mastitis typically occurs 2–6 weeks postpartum; however, 1/3 of cases occur beyond 6 weeks postpartum, often during periods of decreased breast-feeding, since milk stasis is thought to predispose to infection
- Incidence is 2–5% of breast-feeding mothers; >50% of cases seen in primiparas
- Risk factors include maternal fatigue, poor nursing technique, nipple trauma, and epidemic *Staphylococcus aureus*
- Causative organisms include *S. aureus* (most common), *S. epidermidis*, streptococci, and gram-negative rods (rare)
- Organisms are almost always bacterial flora from the nursing infant's nose and throat; they enter the breast through the nipple at the site of a fissure or abrasion, which may be quite small
- Nonpuerperal breast infections are often associated with mammary duct ectasia, tend to be subacute, and tend to have a relapsing course

Differential Dx

- Puerperal mastitis
  - Engorement with milk
  - Obstructed milk duct
  - Trauma
  - Galactocele
  - *Candida albicans* infection
  - Supernumerary breasts
- Nonpuerperal mastitis
  - Trauma
  - Inflammatory breast cancer
  - Fat necrosis
  - Granuloma

Presentation

- Puerperal mastitis
  - Fever
  - Localized erythema
  - Tenderness and induration
  - Palpable heat over affected area
  - Early infection may be simple cellulitis; late may be abscess
  - Associated symptoms include malaise, nausea, flu-like symptoms
- Nonpuerperal mastitis
  - Systemic toxicity is rarely present
  - Localized erythema, point tenderness, and induration of the skin surrounding the nipple
  - Palpable masses and mammographic changes may occur due to chronic inflammation and scarring, mimicking carcinoma

Diagnosis/Evaluation

- Usually a clinical diagnosis based on signs and symptoms
- In puerperal mastitis, milk can be expressed from the affected breast and cultured to identify organisms and antimicrobial sensitivities
- Milk content can be analyzed microscopically to quantify bacteria and leukocytes (leukocytes >10^6/mL or bacteria >10^3/mL signify infection)
- Ultrasound is useful to rule out abscess

Treatment

- Puerperal mastitis
  - Assess nursing technique
  - Prevent nipple damage via pre-feeding manual expression or pumping, correction of latch-on, rotation of positions to minimize trauma, drying with heat, and nipple shield
  - Continue breast-feeding with frequent emptying of the infected breast
  - Antibiotics to cover *S. aureus*, *S. epidermidis*, and streptococci include dicloxacillin or first-generation cephalosporins
- Nonpuerperal mastitis
  - Antibiotic coverage of gram-positive and anaerobic bacteria (e.g., amoxicillin plus clavulanate)
  - Application of moist heat and nipple hygiene with hexachlorophene or povidone-iodine
- Abscess formation requires ultrasound-guided needle aspiration or surgical drainage and appropriate antibiotics

Prognosis/Complications

- Puerperal mastitis
  - With frequent emptying and antibiotics, resolution occurs in 97% of cases
  - With delayed treatment, abscess formation occurs in 10% of cases
  - There is an increased risk of recurrence of mastitis during the same lactation period and with subsequent pregnancies
- Nonpuerperal mastitis
  - Chronic, relapsing infection may require surgical excision of the subareolar duct complex

118. Postpartum Depression

Etiology/Pathophysiology

- Postpartum depression occurs in at least 10% of pregnancies
- Usually begins within 6 weeks of delivery and persists for 3–14 months
- Etiology is unknown; however, most studies show that hormonal imbalance plays a role (levels of estrogen, progesterone, and cortisol fall dramatically within 48 hours after delivery—women who develop postpartum depression may be more sensitive to these hormonal changes)
- Risk factors include a history of prior postpartum depression, major depression, psychosocial stress, and inadequate social support
- There is no association with social class, marital status, or parity
- The "baby blues" is a passing state of heightened emotions that occur in up to 85% of women who have recently given birth; it peaks 3–5 days after delivery and resolves within the first 2 postpartum weeks
- Postpartum psychosis is very rare and occurs within 3 weeks of delivery; may include mania, severe depression, delusions, and/or hallucinations

Differential Dx

- "Baby blues"
- Postpartum psychosis
- Hypothyroidism
- Anemia due to blood loss

Presentation

- Symptoms occur from 24 hours to 6 months following delivery
- Signs and symptoms are indistinguishable from major depression (e.g., sad mood, lack of pleasure or interest, sleep disturbance, weight loss, loss of energy, tearfulness, suicidal thoughts)
- The mother may be ambivalent or have negative feelings toward her child
- The mother may have thoughts or fears about hurting her child

Diagnosis/Evaluation

- Exclude medical causes (e.g., thyroid dysfunction, anemia)
- Initial labs should include thyroid function tests and CBC
- Diagnosis of postpartum depression is based on DSM IV criteria for major depression occurring within 4 weeks of delivery
- The Edinburgh Postnatal Depression Scale (EPDS) is a 10-item self-rated questionnaire used to detect postpartum depression
  - A score of 12 or more on EPDS or an affirmative answer on question 10 (presence of suicidal thoughts) requires a more thorough evaluation

Treatment

- Postpartum blues does not require specific therapy and usually resolves spontaneously
- Optimal treatment includes counseling and medication; pharmacologic therapy (6–12 months duration) is recommended in first episodes
  - SSRIs are first-line therapy
  - Breast-feeding women must be informed that antidepressants are secreted into breast milk; however, serum SSRI levels in the nursing infant are generally low or undetectable
  - Prophylactic SSRIs may be started 2–3 weeks before delivery or at delivery in patients with a prior history of postpartum depression
- Inpatient hospitalization may be necessary for severe postpartum depression

Prognosis/Complications

- Women with a prior history of postpartum depression may have up to a 90% risk of recurrence; prophylactic SSRIs may be started 2–3 weeks prior to delivery or at delivery
- Earlier initiation of treatment is associated with better prognosis
- Postpartum depression may negatively affect the mother-infant interaction
- Children of mothers with postpartum depression are more likely to exhibit behavioral problems, delays in cognitive development, emotional disturbances, and early onset of depressive illness
- Though postpartum psychosis is rare, suicide occurs in 5% and infanticide in 4% of patients with postpartum psychosis

Menopause & Related Disorders

ALEXANDRA BAGERIS
PHYLLIS L. CARR, MD
CLAUDIA DE YOUNG, MD, MSc
ELIZABETH DUPUIS, MD
KAREN M. FREUND, MD, MPH
OMAR MULLA-OSSMAN, MD
MICHELE SINOPOLI, MD
TU-MAI TRAN, MD

119. Well Care of Elderly Women

- At birth, an American female is expected to live 79.5 years; by age 65 she is expected to live another 19.2 years
- Well care includes screening services and therapeutics aimed at preserving health and enhancing function
- The top ten causes of death for women over 65 years are heart disease, influenza and pneumonia, cancer, diabetes mellitus, cerebrovascular disease, renal disease, chronic lower respiratory disease, accident, Alzheimer's disease, septicemia

Blood Pressure
- Measure every 1–2 years
- Treating hypertension reduces age-adjusted coronary artery disease mortality

Nutrition and Physical Activity
- Measure weight and ask about appetite changes
- Counsel regarding a balanced diet and vitamin supplementation – older women should receive at least 800 IU of vitamin D and 1.2 gm of elemental calcium to help prevent osteoporotic fractures
- Encourage the incorporation of physical activity into daily routines

Screening
- Periodic total cholesterol screening for women age 45–65 years
- Screen for subclinical thyroid disease by measuring serum TSH every 5 years after age 55
- Periodic bone density measurements in women over the age of 65 years

Cancer Screening
- Colorectal cancer screening after age 50 with annual fecal occult blood testing, sigmoidoscopy, or both
- Breast cancer screening with mammography every 1–2 years in women 40–69
- Pap test every 1–3 years in all women who are sexually active and have a cervix; consider discontinuation of testing after age 54 if previous regular screening was normal and no new sexual partners

Mental Status/Cognition
- Dementia is prevalent in 20–50% of people over 85 years old
- Screen with Folstein Mini-Mental State exam, and screen for depression

Substance Abuse
- Smoking cessation counseling and CAGE screening for alcohol abuse

Sexuality and Incontinence
- 17–55% of elderly women suffer from incontinence; patients are often reluctant to bring up these issues, so it is important to initiate discussion
- Review medications and chronic conditions that could influence either of these issues

Injury Prevention
- Burn injuries occur more frequently in people over 60 years – counsel regarding the installation of smoke detectors and reducing the water temperature to below 48.8°C (120°F)
- 30% of non-institutionalized elders fall each year – discuss proper lighting, correcting slippery floors and loose rugs, and installing handrails/grab bars
- Counsel safety belt use while driving

Hearing and Vision Screening
- Snellen acuity testing and glaucoma screening every 1–2 years in people over 60 years old
- Assess for hearing impairment periodically

Dental/Oral Care
- Oral cancer screening includes inspection and palpation of the oral cavity, and palpation of head and neck lymph nodes
- Recommend flossing and brushing daily, and recommend visiting the dentist periodically

Advance Directives and Health Care Proxy
- Discuss with patient during health maintenance exam

Immunizations
- Tetanus-diphtheria booster every 10 years
- After age 50, vaccinate against influenza annually and pneumoccocal infection once at 65

120. Perimenopause

Etiology/Pathophysiology

- Perimenopause
  - Begins 2–8 years before menopause
  - Lasts 1 year after the last menstrual period
  - Vasomotor symptoms and irregular menses commence
  - Characterized by normal ovulatory cycles interspersed with anovulatory cycles of varying length
  - Associated with an accelerated rate of oocyte atresia
- Menopause
  - Permanent cessation of menstruation
  - Begins 12 months after the final menses
  - Mean age of onset in U.S. is 51 years
  - Loss of ovarian sensitivity to FSH/LH stimulation
  - Oocyte atresia ultimately results in estrogen deficiency
- Hot flashes are the most common postmenopausal complaint: Sudden onset of reddening and warmth of the skin over the head, neck, and chest, lasting minutes; no inherent health hazard; coincides with an LH surge

Differential Dx

- Premature ovarian failure (menopause before 40 years old)
- Late menopause (after 55 years old)
- Surgical menopause
- Amenorrhea due to pregnancy or endocrine abnormality

Presentation

- Routine health maintenance exam
- Perimenopausal symptoms
  - Dysfunctional uterine bleeding
  - Sleep disturbance
  - Hot flashes
  - Mood lability
- Postmenopausal symptoms
  - Headaches
  - Decreased libido
  - Urogenital changes (vaginal dryness, pruritis, and dyspareunia)
  - Hot flashes

Diagnosis/Evaluation

- Perimenopause is a clinical diagnosis characterized by changes in the menstrual cycle length and symptom level discomfort
- The serum FSH level that is diagnostic of menopause varies depending on the assay used, but is greater than the upper limit of normal for reproductive-age women (~20 IU/L)
- FSH:LH ratio >1
- Given fluctuations in levels, estradiol, LH, and FSH are not helpful in assessing perimenopause and should not be obtained to determine absolute values
- Workup of dysfunctional uterine bleeding
  - Transvaginal ultrasound
  - If endometrium is >4 mm, proceed to office aspiration curettage
  - If unable to perform office curettage, perform in-hospital dilatation and curettage
  - Hysteroscopy or ultrasonography with uterine saline instillation if bleeding persists, to evaluate for polyps or fibroids

Treatment

- Oral contraceptives can be continued through perimenopause for reduction of vasomotor symptoms and control of dysfunctional uterine bleeding; prescribe only to nonsmokers and women without CAD risk factors
- In smokers with irregular menses, progestin may be used to induce monthly withdrawal bleed to regulate menses
- Hormone replacement therapy (see *Hormone Replacement Therapy* entry) is useful for short-term symptomatic treatment
- Some patients may be using natural supplements to treat the symptoms of menopause (e.g., dong quai, black cohosh, soy products); randomized controlled trials have found no benefit from black cohosh and phyto-estrogens compared with placebo
- Hot flashes may be treated with hormone replacement therapy, SSRIs, clonidine
- Urogenital changes may be treated with hormone replacement or topical (vaginal) estrogens

Prognosis/Complications

- Dysfunctional uterine bleeding
  - Unopposed estrogen during perimenopause
  - Endometrial hyperplasia
  - Increased risk for endometrial carcinoma
- Osteoporosis
  - Low bone mass with fractures
  - With declining estrogen, bone remodeling increases
  - Evaluate with bone density studies
  - Calcium and vitamin D supplementation
  - Bisphosphonates
  - Raloxifene
- Hormone replacement therapy
  - Helpful for short-term symptomatic control
  - Slight increased risk of cardiovascular disease and breast cancer (19 additional events per year per 10,000 women)

121. Osteoporosis

Etiology/Pathophysiology

- International consensus definition: Low bone mass and micro-architectural deterioration of bone tissue (i.e., poor bone quality)
- World Health Organization definition is based on bone mineral density, where the T-score is the number of standard deviations below or above the mean bone density for healthy young adults
  - Normal: T-score greater than −1.0
  - Low bone mass (osteopenia): T-score less than −1.0 but greater than −2.5
  - Osteoporosis: T-score −2.5 or less
  - Severe (established) osteoporosis: T-score −2.5 or less in the presence of one or more fragility fractures
- Half of all postmenopausal women will experience an osteoporosis-related fracture
- Nonmodifiable risk factors: Age, female sex, white or Asian, small body frame, family history, surgical menopause, hyperthyroid/parathyroid, and hypogonadism
- Modifiable risk factors: Smoking, alcohol abuse, calcium or vitamin D deficiency, lifetime of inactivity, medications (e.g., anticonvulsants, steroids, chemotherapy, lithium), high caffeine intake

Differential Dx

- Malignancy/tumor
- Paget's disease
- Osteomalacia
- Renal dystrophy
- Ischemic bone disease

Presentation

- Usually asymptomatic; diagnosed from bone mineral density measurement
- Kyphosis indicates multiple fractures
- Back pain due to vertebral fractures
- Fracture after fall (e.g., hip, wrist)
- Consider osteoporosis in patients who have had >1 inch height loss

Diagnosis/Evaluation

- Bone mineral density (BMD) measurement: Preferred test is hip and spine dual-energy photon X-ray absorptiometry (DEXA) scan
- Optional lab tests in healthy women to rule out secondary causes of osteoporosis
  - 24-hour urinary calcium measurement
  - Serum calcium, parathyroid hormone, and 25-hydroxyvitamin D measurements
  - TSH for patients on thyroid replacement medication
  - Urinary n-telopeptide (a marker of bone resorption)

Treatment

- Adequate dietary calcium supplementation (adults: 1,000–1,200 mg/day) is required with all therapies in order to maintain or increase bone mass
- Adequate vitamin D supplementation (400 IU/day) is required with all therapies to ensure adequate absorption of calcium and normal bone production
- Adequate physical activity is essential, especially weight bearing activity; physical activity helps to directly increase bone density, strengthening muscles, and prevent falls
- Avoid tobacco and alcohol abuse
- Pharmacologic agents:
  - Bisphosphonates (e.g., alendronate, risedronate)
  - Raloxifene
  - Estrogen
  - Calcitonin
  - Parathyroid hormone (this is the only treatment that stimulates bone formation)

Prognosis/Complications

- Low bone mass is the most important risk factor for predicting first fracture
- Relative risk for fracture roughly doubles for each standard deviation decrease in bone mineral density
- Osteoporosis-related hip fractures are associated with a 20% increase in mortality in the year following the fracture
- Treatment of osteoporosis with bisphosphonates results in a 30–50% reduction in risk for fractures, depending on site and prior fracture history

122. Urinary Incontinence

Etiology/Pathophysiology

- Affects 15–30% of adults older than 65 (2:1 female-to-male ratio)
- Stress incontinence: Loss of urine associated with a rise in intra-abdominal pressure (e.g., coughing, lifting, bending, exercising)
  - Risk factors include vaginal childbirth, episiotomy, estrogen depletion, genito-urinary surgery/radiation, and chronic cough
- Urge incontinence (overactive bladder): Loss of urine due to hyperactivity of the detrusor muscle
  - Most cases are age-related and idiopathic
  - May occur secondary to loss of cortical inhibition of the micturition reflex (e.g., stroke, Parkinson's disease)
  - Local bladder etiologies include bladder tumors, stones, and infections
- Overflow incontinence: Loss of urine due to excess urine storage, either due to an atonic bladder (e.g., diabetic neuropathy, pelvic surgery, anticholinergic medications, spinal stenosis) or a bladder outlet obstruction (e.g., strictures)
- Physiologic changes of aging predispose, but do not cause, incontinence: Decreased bladder capacity and shortened urethra, increased involuntary bladder muscle contractions, decreased detrusor contractility, decreased mobility and functional capacity

Differential Dx

- Reversible diagnoses ("**DIAPERS**")
  - **D**elirium/dementia
  - **I**nfection
  - **A**trophic vaginitis
  - **P**harmaceuticals
  - **E**xcess urine output
  - **R**estricted mobility
  - **S**tool
- Functional incontinence (impaired mobility)
- Vesicovaginal fistula

Presentation

- Stress incontinence: History of incontinence following maneuvers that increase intra-abdominal pressure (e.g., coughing, lifting, bending, exercising)
- Urge incontinence: Patient is unable to sustain continence due to frequent urges to void ("cannot get to toilet in time")
- Overflow incontinence: Patient notices voiding small volumes of urine and notices bladder is full even after voiding (e.g., feeling of fullness, increased abdominal girth, suprapubic discomfort)
- Excoriation/skin care issues

Diagnosis/Evaluation

- History should focus on precipitating symptoms, frequency, volume, timing, urge symptoms, bowel function, fluid intake, medications, and prior pelvic and abdominal surgery
- Physical examination should include alertness and functional status, leakage with Valsalva maneuver, and neurologic evaluation; filling the bladder prior to exam is helpful
  - Abdomen: Percuss for bladder distension and tenderness
  - Pelvic: Observe for atrophy, loss of urine upon coughing, cystocele and rectocele, motion at bladder neck, and masses
  - Rectal: Evaluate for fecal impaction and masses
  - CNS: Evaluate for peri-anal sensation, lower extremity weakness, and spinal cord defect or stenosis
- Labs should include a urinalysis, blood glucose, calcium, BUN/creatinine, vitamin B_{12}, RPR, and urine culture
- Post-void residual can be evaluated by catheterization or ultrasound; elevated (>100 cc) in overflow incontinence
- Cystoscopy is indicated for hematuria or persistent pyuria to rule out tumor or fistula
- Fluorourodynamic testing is indicated in difficult cases

Treatment

- Stress incontinence is generally treated surgically to elevate and suspend the bladder and bladder neck
  - Kegel exercises, pessary for bladder or uterine prolapse, and urethral collagen injections may help
  - Medical treatments include α-adrenergics, anticholinergics, and estrogen creams
  - Surgical options include pubovaginal sling or transvaginal suspension
- Urge incontinence is generally treated medically
  - Anticholinergics (e.g., oxybutynin, tolterodine) are often effective to improve detrusor instability
  - Other treatments include bladder re-training (timed voiding), prompted voiding, biofeedback, and sacral nerve stimulators
- Overflow incontinence: Reduce bladder fullness by prompted voiding, bladder decompression via intermittent catheterizations, cholinergic medications (e.g., bethanechol), or nerve stimulators

Prognosis/Complications

- Involuntary loss of urine afflicts millions and is associated with significant psychological morbidity and social impairment
- Although urinary incontinence is a very common chronic condition, few women seek medical attention
- Stress incontinence: Sling procedures are successful in >80% of cases
- Urge incontinence: Medical management is successful in >80% of cases
- Overflow incontinence: If not managed properly, may lead to renal failure
- Complications include local skin infection (cellulitis, peri-anal candida infection, ulcers), urinary tract infection, urosepsis, psychological issues (social isolation, depression, sexual and sleep dysfunction)

123. Pelvic Prolapse

Etiology/Pathophysiology

- Weakening pelvic floor muscle/fascia matrix results in displacement of organs (e.g., uterus, bladder, rectum) from their normal anatomic position
- Common in young and elderly women—incidence is 30–50%
- Pelvic organs are attached to the bony pelvis by the levator ani muscles, neurovascular system, and connective tissue (uterosacral/cardinal ligament complex and endopelvic fascia)
- Risk factors include multiparity (large infant, long or difficult labor), obesity, pelvic surgery, connective tissue disease, neurologic dysfunction, chronic constipation or cough, strenuous exercise, and estrogen deficiency
- May occur following childbirth (due to stretching of tissue) and with menopause (due to weakened and less elastic ligaments)
- The site of muscle or fascia damage determines the type of prolapse
  - Cystocele (anterior vaginal wall defect): Downward displacement of bladder
  - Rectocele (posterior vaginal wall defect): Protrusion of the rectum into the posterior vaginal lumen
  - Enterocele (posterior vaginal wall defect): Small bowel presses into vagina
  - Uterine/vaginal vault prolapse: Forward dislocation of uterus and cervix toward the introitus

Differential Dx

- Cystocele
- Rectocele
- Enterocele
- Uterine/vaginal vault prolapse

Presentation

- Mild prolapse is asymptomatic, and often found incidentally on exam
- Cystocele and cystourethrocele: Difficulty emptying bladder, stress urinary incontinence, and dyspareunia
- Rectocele and enterocele: Constipation, difficulty completing bowel movement (manual pressure is required to evacuate rectum), fecal incontinence, and dyspareunia
- Uterine/vaginal vault prolapse: Feeling of pressure or mass in vagina, back pain, painful intercourse, and visible protruding bulge

Diagnosis/Evaluation

- History should include history of vaginal deliveries or prior pelvic surgery, menopause status, onset of symptoms, characteristics, precipitants, and any associated urinary incontinence
- Site-specific exam of vagina with single-blade speculum for 3-dimensional defect of vaginal wall (retract the anterior, posterior, and lateral walls); exam should occur both supine and standing, with and without Valsalva, and with digital retrovaginal exam (for rectocele)
- Staging systems are used clinically to assess the degree of prolapse
  - The Pelvic Organ Prolapse Staging System measures (in centimeters) the positions of nine sites of the vagina and the perineal body in relationship to the hymen
  - The Baden grading system includes grade 0 (no prolapse), grade 1 (prolapse halfway to the hymen), grade 2 (prolapse to the introitus), grade 3 (prolapse halfway beyond the hymen), and grade 4 (complete prolapse)

Treatment

- Asymptomatic prolapse requires only preventive lifestyle modifications: Kegel exercises to strengthen the pelvic muscles, smoking cessation, weight loss, and avoidance of increases in intra-abdominal pressure (e.g., constipation, straining, or strenuous activities)
- Nonsurgical interventions for symptomatic prolapse include lifestyle modifications (as above), hormone therapy, and use of pessary (temporary or permanent)
- Pelvic reconstructive surgery may be indicated
  - Cystocele: Anterior colporrhaphy or transvaginal paravaginal repair (occasionally with surgical correction of urinary incontinence)
  - Rectocele: Posterior colporrhaphy, grafting, or rectal wall imbrication
  - Vaginal vault prolapse: Colpectomy/colpocleisis or colpopexy (preserves sexual function)
  - Uterine prolapse: Hysterectomy
- Radiotherapy may be used to shorten fascia/muscles

Prognosis/Complications

- Pelvic prolapse can be a significant, debilitating health problem that interferes with daily function and quality of life
- Women may not be aware of the extent of damage, are too embarrassed to seek medical attention, or attribute it to aging
- Surgical repair of prolapse, depending on technique and severity of the defect, has a 65–90% success rate
- Extensive postoperative care and adherence to lifestyle modifications is necessary
- Postoperative complications include strictures (due to excessive trimming), fecal and urinary fistulas, dyspareunia and sexual dysfunction (due to overzealous tightening), vaginal granulation, and scarring

124. Hormone Replacement Therapy

Indications

- Menopausal symptoms, including hot flashes, vaginal atrophy and dryness, mood difficulties, and sleep difficulties (insomnia, night sweats)
- Osteoporosis and fracture prevention
- *Not* to be used for primary or secondary prevention of cardiovascular disease, stroke, or dementia
- Estrogen/progesterone combination treatment can be continuous or cyclic (cyclic is cyclic progesterone with continuous estrogen)
  - Continuous: For women clearly in menopause no menses is triggered
  - Cyclic: For women just entering menopause with oligomenorrhea; a monthly menses is triggered, erratic spotting avoided, and can switch to continuous preparation in a year
- Estrogen and progesterone most commonly given as oral formulation; patch is available for estrogen, but no clear advantage
- Trend is toward short-term use (<3 years) at the lowest effective dose
- Vaginal estrogen formulations are available (cream or delivery systems) and are useful for vaginal or urethral atrophy; do not require progesterone

Epidemiology

- Eligible patients
  - Menopause symptoms
  - Osteoporosis (if other treatments are not indicated)
- Ineligible patients
  - History of DVT or thromboembolism
  - History of cardiac disease and/or stroke
  - History of breast cancer or high risk of breast cancer
  - Undiagnosed abnormal vaginal bleeding
  - Pregnancy
  - Liver disease

Side Effects

- Vaginal bleeding/spotting: Must be addressed if heavy or frequent; requires further evaluation to rule out endometrial pathology if mild spotting persists beyond 3–6 months
- Hormones may trigger migraines in some women, but ameliorate them in others
- Breast discomfort
- Bloating
- Endometriosis exacerbation
- Micronized progesterone may cause fewer side effects than medroxyprogesterone

Alternative Treatments

- Hot flashes: Venlafaxine, clonidine, SSRIs; progestins also are effective but cause weight gain
- Soy products and other botanicals have not been shown in trials to provide benefit over placebo
- Vaginal atrophy: Vaginal estrogen; water or glycerin-based lubricants
- Mood and sleep difficulties: SSRIs, trazodone
- Osteoporosis: Bisphosphonates, raloxifene

Efficacy

- Menopausal symptoms: Initial effects within days to weeks, full effect within 8–12 weeks
- Osteoporosis prevention effects seen in 1–2 years
- The routine use of estrogen and progestin for the prevention of chronic conditions (heart disease, stroke, Alzheimer's) is not recommended

Complications

- Venous thromboembolic events
- Cardiac event
- Stroke
- Breast cancer
- All women with a uterus *must* have progesterone to oppose oral estrogen effects on the uterus and avoid increased risk of uterine/endometrial cancer
  - If cycling, progesterone for >12 days per month is necessary
  - For vaginal preparations, progesterone is not necessary
- Gallbladder disease
- *Stop* hormone therapy after acute events such as MI, DVT, and prior to surgery or immobilization

125. Heart Disease

Etiology/Pathophysiology

- Atherosclerotic heart disease is a spectrum of disease with narrowed coronary arteries, cholesterol plaques, and fibrotic tissue in the vascular intima
- Results in angina, myocardial infarction (MI), and congestive heart disease (CHF)
- Epidemiology
  - Women's risk of heart disease increases two-fold after menopause
  - Peak incidence is age 60–70
  - Cardiovascular disease kills more women than any other disease and accounts for 45% of all deaths in women
- Risk factors in women include diabetes mellitus, hypertension, tobacco, total cholesterol >240 mg/dL, HDL <35 mg/dL, sedentary lifestyle, obesity, family history with MI before age 60, age >55 years, and black or Hispanic race
- Oral contraceptive pill use is known to increase the risk of acute MI in women who smoke and/or are hypertensive; however, there is no evidence of increased risk in women without risk factors

Differential Dx

- GI disease: Gastric ulcer, esophagitis, gastroesophageal reflux, cholecystitis
- Pulmonary embolism
- Chest wall disease: Costochondritis, herpes zoster, thrombophlebitis
- Lung disease: Pleuritis, pleural adhesions, pneumothorax
- Infectious cardiomyopathy
- Aortic aneurysm
- Pericarditis
- Mitral valve prolapse

Presentation

- Substernal chest pain
- Dyspnea on exertion
- Paroxysmal nocturnal dyspnea
- Orthopnea
- Edema
- Murmur
- Women are more likely than men to be asymptomatic or present with atypical symptoms during MI
- Atypical symptoms of acute MI include nausea, vomiting, fatigue, and malaise

Diagnosis/Evaluation

- Laboratory studies for the diagnosis of MI include elevation of cardiac enzymes (CPK, CPK isoenzymes, SGOT, LDH, troponin)
- Serum risk factors include elevated triglycerides, cholesterol, LDL, glucose, and hemoglobinA_{IC}; decreased HDL
- EKG may reveal ST segment depression or elevation and/or T wave inversion
- Exercise EKG stress testing has low cost and has been shown to be effective in women
- Exercise echocardiography may reveal wall motion abnormalities; more sensitive and specific for CAD than exercise EKG
- Pharmacologic stress echocardiography is useful in women who are not able to exercise
- Angiography may reveal narrowing of coronary arteries (significant stenosis is >75%)
- Cardiac catheterization

Treatment

- Prevent further progression of disease by treating hypercholesterolemia and controlling blood pressure and diabetes; initial management of these conditions includes encouraging dietary modification, regular exercise, and smoking cessation
- Hormone replacement therapy: The use of estrogen and progestin are not effective in primary or secondary prevention of heart disease
- Women benefit from use of aspirin and β-blockers for secondary preventive therapy
- Thrombolytics must be used cautiously as women have a higher risk of stroke and hemorrhage than in men
- Revascularization: Due to the smaller size of women's vessels, there is a higher technical failure rate in women than in men

Prognosis/Complications

- Long-term prognosis depends on severity of underlying disease and the patient's co-morbidities
- Complications include MI, CHF, arrhythmias and sudden death
- Women tend to present with more advanced CAD than men
- Women who suffer MI are three times as likely to die from the ischemic event or complications than their male counterparts
- Yentl syndrome: Women with undocumented coronary artery disease are treated less aggressively than men (women have lower rates of hospitalization and cardiac catheterization); however, heart disease and MI in women are as significant a health risk as in men

126. Stroke

Etiology/Pathophysiology

- Third leading cause of death in women
- Risk factors include hypertension, diabetes, smoking, atrial fibrillation, OCP use, history of TIA, hypercholesterolemia
- Ischemic strokes constitute 85% of all strokes
  - Embolic strokes: Cardiogenic (e.g., atrial fibrillation, mural thrombosis, endocarditis), artery-to-artery (atherothrombosis displaced distally), embolus secondary to a hypercoagulable state (e.g., SLE, protein C or S deficiency), paradoxical embolus through a patent foramen ovale
  - Lacunar strokes: Chronic hypertension damages the endothelium of the brain's penetrating small vessels, causing progressive occlusion (lipohyalinosis); results in lacunar syndromes (e.g., pure unilateral motor or sensory deficits, dysarthria, clumsy-hand syndrome, ataxic hemiparesis)
- Hemorrhagic strokes constitute 15% of all strokes
  - Parenchymal: Rupture of penetrating blood vessels due to hypertension (putamin, thalamus, pons, cerebellum), tumor, amyloidosis
  - Subdural: Tearing of dural bridging veins secondary to head trauma
  - Epidural: Injury to middle meningeal artery secondary to a skull fracture
  - Subarachnoid: Due to aneurysm rupture, arteriovenous malformation, trauma

Differential Dx

- Transient ischemic attack
- Brain tumor
- Todd's paralysis (postictal phenomena)
- Aura of migraine
- Multiple sclerosis
- Brain abscess
- Toxic metabolic encephalopathy
- Encephalitis
- Hypoglycemia (may mimic a new stroke or make an old stroke appear symptomatic again)
- Psychogenic

Presentation

- Ischemic stroke symptoms depend on vascular distribution
  - Anterior cerebral artery (ACA): Contralateral leg weakness, urinary incontinence, gaze deviation
  - Middle cerebral artery (MCA): Contralateral hemiparesis, aphasia, neglect, dysphagia
  - Vertebrobasilar artery: Diplopia, hemianopia, ataxia, hemiparesis, nausea, vertigo
- Hemorrhagic stroke symptoms
  - Sudden onset of severe headache (patients with subarachnoid hemorrhage may report "worst headache of life")
  - Nuchal rigidity, photophobia, nausea, vomiting, focal deficits, lethargy, and seizures may occur

Diagnosis/Evaluation

- Complete history and physical examination
- MRI of the brain can detect a new ischemic stroke within about 2 hours of onset (changes on CT take >24 hrs to appear)
- Magnetic resonant angiogram (MRA) of the brain may detect blood vessel narrowing, dissection, and some aneurysms
- Diffusion weighted images (DWI) of the brain are sensitive to detect the location of acute ischemic brain tissue
- Transthoracic echocardiogram (TTE) may be used to detect cardiogenic embolus; however, TEE is more sensitive
- Carotid duplex screening for carotid occlusive disease
- Transcranial Doppler (TCD) will evaluate MCA circulation
- Cerebral angiogram is gold standard to detect aneurysms
- ECG may reveal atrial fibrillation as a source of emboli
- EEG may show focal slowing if cortex is involved
- Laboratory testing for young women may include CBC, anticardiolipin, Lupus anticoagulant, antithrombin III, ANA, ESR, ANC, factor V Leiden, C-reactive protein, homocysteine, HbA_{IC}, and a lipid panel

Treatment

- Treatment depends largely on the stroke etiology
  - Anticoagulation is indicated for atrial fibrillation, impending carotid or basilar occlusion, mural thrombosis, patent foramen ovale with mural aneurysm, and women who test positive for lupus anticoagulant with antiphospholipid antibodies
  - Lacunar infarcts are treated with antiplatelet therapy (e.g., aspirin)
  - Vasculitis (e.g., temporal arteritis) is treated with steroids
  - Endocarditis is treated with antibiotics
  - Arteriovenous malformations may require resection
  - Aneurysms are often treated surgically
  - Endarterectomy is effective in patients with critical unilateral or bilateral carotid stenosis (rates of endarterectomy are lower in women, but aggressive management of strokes are equally effective in women as in men)

Prognosis/Complications

- 47% of strokes in pregnancy are ischemic
  - 80% result from arterial occlusion (increased in second and third trimester)
  - 20% result from central venous occlusion (increased in first trimester)
  - Risks for embolism include fibromuscular dysplasia, sickle cell, antiphospholipid antibodies, antithrombin III or protein C&S deficiency
- Hemorrhagic strokes in pregnancy: 44% of strokes in pregnancy; usually result from eclampsia
- Oral contraceptives and smoking increase risk
- Estradiol replacement in menopausal women has no value in stroke prevention
- Prognosis depends on size and area of stroke

Index

Index

Index

Index

Female adolescents, well care of, 2
Female sexual dysfunction (FSD), 40
Fetal abnormality, as differential diagnosis, 128
Fetal aneuploidy, 91
Fetal bradycardia, as differential diagnosis, 127
Fetal CNS abnormalities, as differential diagnosis, 106
Fetal death, 108
Fetal genetic abnormalities, as differential diagnosis, 108
Fetal growth restriction, 103
Fetal growth restriction, as differential diagnosis, 105
Fetal heart failure, as differential diagnosis, 107
Fetal heart rate monitoring (FHR), 114
Fetal hypoxia, as differential diagnosis, 105
Fetal malpresentations, as differential diagnosis, 128
Fetal physiology, 89
Fetal urinary abnormalities, as differential diagnosis, 105
Fetal vessel rupture, 102
Feto-maternal hemorrhage, as differential diagnosis, 107
Fibroadenoma, as differential diagnosis, 30, 49
Fibrocystic breast changes, as differential diagnosis, 49
Fibroids, 29
Fibroids, as differential diagnosis, 28, 41, 42, 94
Fibromyalgia, as differential diagnosis, 24
Fitz-Hugh-Curtis syndrome, as differential diagnosis, 66
Follicular cyst, as differential diagnosis, 50, 51
Folliculitis, as differential diagnosis, 33, 56
Footling or hand presentation, 126, 127
Foreign object, as differential diagnosis, 22
Functional incontinence, as differential diagnosis, 141
Functional ovarian cysts, 25
Furunculosis, as differential diagnosis, 33
Galactocele, as differential diagnosis, 134
Galactorrhea, 31
Gallbladder disease, 66
Gallbladder disease, as differential diagnosis, 75
Gamete intrafallopian transfer (GIFT), 43
Gardnerella vaginalis, in bacterial vaginosis, 32
Gastric ulcer, as differential diagnosis, 144
Gastritis, as differential diagnosis, 66
Gastroenteritis, as differential diagnosis, 97
Gastroesophageal reflux disease (GERD), as differential diagnosis, 63, 144
Genetic defects, as differential diagnosis, 72
Genetic syndromes, as differential diagnosis, 72, 103, 104
Genital tract lesion, as differential diagnosis, 95
Genital trauma, as differential diagnosis, 37
Genital warts, as differential diagnosis, 34
Gestational diabetes mellitus (DM), as differential diagnosis, 104
Gestational diabetes mellitus (GDM), 73
Gestational hypertension, 98

Gestational hypertension, as differential diagnosis, 75, 98
Gestational trophoblastic disease, as differential diagnosis, 95
Gestational trophoblastic neoplasia (GTN), 57
Giant cell arteritis, as differential diagnosis, 68
Glaucoma, as differential diagnosis, 68
Glomerulonephritis, as differential diagnosis, 75
Glucagonoma, as differential diagnosis, 72
Glucose intolerance, as differential diagnosis, 73
Gonadal dysgenesis, as differential diagnosis, 23
Gonorrhea, as differential diagnosis, 32, 34, 60
Granuloma, as differential diagnosis, 134
Granuloma inguinale, as differential diagnosis, 37
Graves' disease, 64
Gravid uterus, as differential diagnosis, 29
Group A Streptococcus, in URIs, 61
Group B Streptococcus
    in C-section wound infections, 133
    in PID, 35
    in postpartum endometritis, 131
Group C Streptococcus, in URIs, 61
Gynecologic and preventive care, 7-17
Gynecologic oncology, 47-57
    breast cancer screening, 10
    cervical cancer screening, 11
    endometrial cancer screening, 12
    ovarian cancer screening, 12

Haemophilus influenzae
    in lower respiratory tract infections, 62
    in URIs, 61
Hashimoto's disease, as differential diagnosis, 65
Headache, 68
HEADS assessment, 2, 3
Heart disease, 144
Heart failure, as differential diagnosis, 109
Hematological changes with pregnancy, as differential diagnosis, 48
Hematoma, as differential diagnosis, 133
Hemolytic-uremic syndrome, as differential diagnosis, 98
Hemorrhage, as differential diagnosis, 62, 130
Hemorrhagic corpus luteum, as differential diagnosis, 28
Hemorrhagic cyst, as differential diagnosis, 24
Hemorrhagic pancreatitis, as differential diagnosis, 100
Hemorrhagic stroke, 145
Hemorrhoids, as differential diagnosis, 48, 102
Hepatitis, as differential diagnosis, 66, 97
Hepatitis A, adult immunization for, 8, 9
Hepatitis B, adult immunization for, 8, 9
Herpes, as differential diagnosis, 32
Herpes simplex virus (HSV), 37
    as differential diagnosis, 34
    in vulvar disease, 33

Index

Index

Index

Index

Index